A Beacon Of Hope For Adolescent Depression

PARENT HANDBOOK ON
CHILDHOOD AND TEEN
DEPRESSION

SECOND EDITION

w: www.erikaslighthouse.org
e: info@erikaslighthouse.org

Erika's Lighthouse is a not-for-profit organization dedicated to raising awareness about childhood and teenage depression and mental health. For more information, please visit us at *www.erikaslighthouse.org.*

PARENT HANDBOOK ON CHILDHOOD AND TEEN DEPRESSION SECOND EDITION
ISBN: 978-1-48356-823-2

The photography in this handbook is being used for illustrative purposes only; any person depicted in the photography is a model.

This handbook is based on the experiences of parents dealing with childhood and teenage depression. It was written for parents who are in similar situations. While Erika's Lighthouse consulted with clinical, therapeutic, legal and child development experts when developing this material, it makes no representations about the medical or psychological opinions expressed herein, nor does it accept responsibility for any actions taken as a result of the material or information contained in the handbook. Every child's and family's situation is unique, and Erika's Lighthouse urges parents to seek and find competent professional advice tailored to their own family's situation.

Printed in the United States

Welcome to the *Erika's Lighthouse Parent Handbook on Childhood and Teen Depression, Second Edition*. You may be reading our handbook because you think your child is depressed and you want to know what to do. **We are here to help you.**

you are
not alone

Somewhere between 15 and 20 percent of our children and teens will suffer from at least one depressive episode before they reach adulthood. These episodes come in many forms—ranging from the child who doesn't want to go to school to the teen who is constantly in a rage to the withdrawn child who barely speaks.

Often, these episodes are seen as just a phase, or typical behavior, but depression, clinical depression, is not part of typical behavior—it is a disorder that deserves attention and needs treatment.

Most children and teens who suffer from depression go undiagnosed and untreated. Many parents don't know the signs of depression or where to turn for help, and, if they reach out for help, they often become frustrated trying to find it. Understanding exactly what's going on with your child, finding the right treatment, dealing with the schools—all have their unique challenges and can deplete the energy of even the most dedicated parent.

We hope this handbook will be a helpful guide to you as you deal with the many issues you will likely confront over the course of your child's depression. We know this is probably a frightening time. You may feel helpless and alone. We invite you to read our handbook with the hope that it will give you both some comfort and some answers.

And we hope you will find some helpful tips on how to help your child maintain good mental health and find happiness, something we all want for our children.

Please keep in mind—this is a parent-to-parent guide. It was written by parents, not professionals, and errs on the side of practical, rather than professional, advice. It is not a substitute for professional help, which we urge you to seek. And, of course, we don't have all the solutions. We merely hope that we have at least a few suggestions that will be of some practical help to you.

OUR HANDBOOK IS ORGANIZED INTO THREE SECTIONS

Section One is the practical guide—it will give you suggestions on what to do and how to do it. We put this section first because you may need to plunge right into ideas that you can put into action immediately.

Section Two is a primer—it includes the things you might want to know about depression, mental health care professionals and potential treatments. This is the more textbook-like section of our handbook, and is designed to be read when you are ready to know more about the details and the kinds of help available.

Section Three is about happiness and strategies you and your child can use to foster and maintain good mental health.

Once again, our goal is to help you navigate a difficult time in your life. We hope our handbook will be helpful along your journey. With that in mind, we begin.

a few facts about depression

There is a lot of stigma attached to having depression—as a society we just don't like to talk about it. We feel guilty and ashamed—about having it, even about having it in our family. But the simple fact is that depression is an identifiable and observable disorder with specific symptoms and, like any physical illness you or your child might have, depression should be treated.

EXACTLY WHAT IS DEPRESSION?

First and foremost, depression is a medical term that defines a specific disorder of the brain. It's more than just a sad or depressed mood, which all of us feel from time to time.

Depression, called Major Depression or Major Depressive Disorder by mental health professionals, is a sustained depressed mood, feeling of sadness, loss of interest or pleasure in most activities, sense of worthlessness and/or guilt, and difficulty with concentration, thinking and making decisions.

Some people with depression, especially teens, feel irritable as well. Cognitive symptoms (a drop in grades or difficulty paying attention or making decisions) often appear first.

Frequently, and especially in children and teenagers, these psychological symptoms are accompanied by physical symptoms which can include agitation, fatigue, changes in sleeping patterns, appetite and/or weight, slowed speech and movement, headache, stomach-ache and other aches and pains.

Some depressions are mild and one can function somewhat normally. Some are severe, limiting even the most routine daily activities or leading to thoughts of death or attempts at suicide.

Most depressions last for seven to nine months, though some last longer than that.

Those who suffer from an episode of depression are at a higher risk of having other, usually more severe, episodes during their lifetime. Early onset, such as childhood or adolescence, is often a sign that an episode will recur.

The use of alcohol can increase the risk of depression.

Roughly two-thirds of children and teenagers with depression have another mental disorder. Dysthymia (see Section Two), anxiety disorders, conduct disorder, substance-related disorders, ADHD (attention deficit-hyperactivity disorder) and learning disorders are the most common co-occurring disorders.

Somewhere between 15 and 20% of our youth will suffer from at least one depressive episode before they reach adulthood, and teens suffer from higher rates of depression than do children. *That's too many of our young people suffering,* and, as we noted before, *most go undiagnosed and untreated.*

Our mothers told us to get a good night's sleep, eat healthily and get plenty of exercise and sun—and they were right. These common-sense ideas can help reduce the symptoms of depression.

Research also confirms the benefits of relaxation techniques such as meditation and breathing exercises.

There is good research evidence that we can relieve the symptoms of depressive episodes through treatment—talk therapy, and if that is not effective or the symptoms are severe, talk therapy and medication together.

We discuss depression in more detail in Section Two, but we wanted at least to set the stage for why you should consider having your child assessed and treated if you think he is suffering from depression. And so we move on to just that subject—getting help.

READING OUR HANDBOOK. For ease of reading, we use "he" to refer to your child and "she" to refer to doctors, therapists, teachers, etc. Please indulge us with this convention as you read.

where to begin

It's normal for parents who think their child is suffering from depression to wonder whether they should just wait and see or whether they should seek help.

The symptoms of depression (page 4) are often evident, but sometimes they can be vague and confusing. Both children and their parents often ask themselves: is this depression or just a phase? Sometimes children and teens hide their feelings from their parents and even from themselves.

If you think something is amiss, trust your instinct. If you are unsure, ask a close friend or family member their opinion. The bottom line is, don't hesitate. It's better to err on the side of caution than to wait—and possibly watch your child become increasingly depressed. Increasingly severe depression can be serious.

Your first phone call should be to your child's physician. Why? Family physicians see thousands of children over their years of practice and are good at determining whether or not there is an issue that needs treatment.

The physician should ask to see your child for a physical examination and to run some tests to make sure that nothing else is wrong; some illnesses, like diabetes, thyroid disease and adrenal gland disease, can act like depression and need to be ruled out.

Not all physicians are trained to look for mood disorders like depression, so before you visit the doctor, take some time to jot down your concerns—moods, behaviors and physical symptoms you are seeing in your child:

[ ] I think there is a problem because _____ .
[ ] I heard my child say _____ .
[ ] I saw my child do _____ .
[ ] My child is feeling _____ .
[ ] This is not my child's normal behavior because _____ .
[ ] I've seen this change in my child over the past _____ weeks or _____ months.

Is this an emergency? If your child is in imminent danger of hurting himself or another person, is hearing voices, or is seeing things that aren't there, he may need an immediate evaluation at a hospital.

Either go directly to your hospital or call 9-1-1 for help. Call your child's physician and/or therapist on the way to the hospital to tell her what's going on and get her advice.

Keep a journal. Possibly the best piece of advice we can give at the outset is to keep a journal. You can start the journal by including the notes that you took to the doctor, any test results from your visit, behaviors, moods and physical symptoms you are seeing at home or hearing about from school, and changes in your child's relationships with family members and friends.

Try to keep up with it regularly—it will be a great aid to refer to as your child goes through his treatment.

You may also wish to talk to your child about why you are in contact with the doctor:

[ ] I notice _____ .
[ ] I care about you.
[ ] It's not your fault.
[ ] We will work together to find you help.
[ ] You deserve to feel better.

If the doctor agrees with you that there is a problem, she may offer to prescribe medication to see if that helps alleviate the symptoms. While this may seem to be an easy way to proceed, it's best to see a professional—someone who specializes in mental health—to get a formal mental health assessment. Just as the doctor needs to rule out diseases that act like depression, so someone trained in the field of mental health needs to determine exactly what's going on with your child. Proper treatment depends on an accurate diagnosis.

WHAT IS A MENTAL HEALTH ASSESSMENT?

A mental health assessment is one or a series of interviews and tests designed to give you [1] a diagnosis, and [2] a treatment plan. Often mental health assessments are reasonably simple—one session can be sufficient to give you a working diagnosis and treatment plan. Sometimes a more complete evaluation is needed. If your child's behavior or mood is severe, you may need a formal assessment—a battery of tests—which might include:

[ ] Interviews with and questionnaires for your child, you and other family members
[ ] Interviews with mental health professionals who have worked with your child and/or your family
[ ] Psychological testing of your child's emotional and cognitive functioning
[ ] Neuropsychological testing of your child's thinking and information-processing capabilities
[ ] Psycho-social assessments of your child's interactions with others
[ ] A review of school records, such as report cards
[ ] An evaluation of family dynamics
[ ] A medical evaluation, which could include blood tests and neurological testing of the brain (an EEG and/or MRI).

FOR EASE OF READING, we use the term "therapist" in our handbook to refer to all four mental health professions. In reality, this term and the term "psychotherapist" generally refer to someone who does talk therapy—a psychologist, social worker or counselor. A psychiatrist is referred to simply as a psychiatrist.

HOW DO YOU FIND SOMEONE TO DO THE ASSESSMENT?

Mental health assessments are done by people who specialize in mental health—psychiatrists, psychologists, social workers and counselors. The mental health field is generally one of individual practitioners or small groups of professionals working together, so, like finding physicians, most people find someone to do an assessment by asking people they know—friends, neighbors, other parents, school personnel and members of the clergy—for referrals.

Psychiatrists and psychologists generally have more formal training in assessment than social workers and counselors—if your child has a complicated or severe illness, you may want to have the assessment done by one of these two professionals.

Your child's physician is probably the easiest way to find a therapist to do an assessment for your child. She also may be able to help you get an appointment—practices are often booked well in advance and it can be very helpful to have someone open a door for you.

Taking the extra step to get an assessment may seem unnecessary—you may, understandably, want to get your child directly into therapy. But, taking the time up front to get an assessment may pay off in the long run.

In addition to getting referrals from your child's physician, school or people you know, you can call a local mental health social service agency, hospital or clinic. Many of these institutions perform assessments, often at reduced rates.

If, however, you are waiting for an assessment and your child is getting worse, it might be best to get your child into therapy immediately (see the next section) and come back to the assessment later if the treatment is not working or if you believe the diagnosis you received is not correct.

The Internet can also be of help. Many mental health professional organizations have options on their websites to help you find a therapist in your area. Here are some that may be helpful:

[ ] The American Academy of Child and Adolescent Psychiatry (*www.aacap.org*)

[ ] American Mental Health Counselors Association (*www.amhca.org*)

[ ] The American Psychological Association (*www.apa.org*)

[ ] The Depression and Bipolar Support Alliance (*www.dbsalliance.org*)

[ ] Good Therapy (*www.goodtherapy.org*)

[ ] The National Association of Social Workers (*www.socialworkers.org*)

[ ] The National Board for Certified Counselors (*www.nbcc.org*)

[ ] Psych Central (*www.psychcentral.com*)

[ ] Psychology Today (*www.psychologytoday.com*)

[ ] SAMHSA's Behavorial Treatment Finder (*www.samhsa.gov*)

You will see all sorts of therapists and tempting programs on the Internet. As with all information on the Internet, it's best to check references before embracing a particular therapist or program.

A good use of the Internet is to use trusted websites to compile a preliminary list of potential therapists, and then cull that list using personal references you have received from friends, neighbors, educators and other professionals in your community.

Whichever source you use, it's important to find someone to do the assessment who has seen a wide variety of cases, who has a broad depth of experience at diagnosing mental disorders, and who has experience working with children who are similar in age to your child.

A FEW THINGS TO NOTE ABOUT ASSESSMENTS

Depression and similar disorders are not always easy to diagnose. It's sometimes difficult to tell which disorder is present, and it can often take several sessions to make a correct diagnosis. As we noted before, many children and teenagers with depression also suffer from another mental disorder.

Cognitive symptoms (a drop in grades, difficulty paying attention or making decisions) are often the first symptoms to appear. This may be why depression is sometimes misdiagnosed as a learning disability.

Some disorders can look like depression, but they are not. A good example of this is bipolar disorder. It's very similar to depression until a manic (overly excited or euphoric state) cycle sets in, but it may be several sessions before the manic cycle presents itself to the therapist so that she can accurately identify it.

Diagnosing children is tricky. Children and teenagers—especially children—are often unable to verbalize their feelings—they may not be at a developmental stage that allows them to recognize their feelings and put them into words. Also, children and teenagers are growing rapidly, both physically and mentally. Their moods and behaviors—the manifestations of the disorder—may change along with their growth. Furthermore, some behavior is appropriate at one age, and not another (think temper tantrums)—but children and teenagers can vary greatly from the norm in their developmental stages.

A good diagnostician should consider all of these factors. She should look at whether the symptoms are occurring with unusual frequency, lasting for an abnormal length of time, or occurring at an unexpected time during your child's development. Taking all of these factors into account during the assessment is important because the treatment plan will depend on them.

COMPLETING THE ASSESSMENT

When your child has completed his assessment, it's a good idea to meet with the therapist to discuss the diagnosis and talk about treatment. If there is a report, get a copy of it and read it. It should include both a diagnosis and treatment plan. Write down questions that you have. Here are some to think about:

[ ] How did you arrive at the diagnosis? How certain are you of it?

[ ] Can you tell me about the disorder? What are its symptoms? What is its usual course? Where can I get more information about it?

[ ] Can you tell me about the treatment plan you propose? How does it work? Is this the usual treatment plan for this illness (if not, why did you choose it)? What are the benefits? What are the risks? Are there alternatives? How much time is usually involved in treatment? Is it supported by research? Where can I get more information about the treatment plan and the current research on it?

Involve your child. Ask him to attend the meeting with you. Often, children go through testing, but aren't told what the results of the tests are. If you include your child in the process, he will be better able to understand that it's not "him"— that it's the disorder making him feel the way he does. This can be an important step towards him learning to take ownership of and manage his depression.

In the end, if you don't feel comfortable with the diagnosis, or are unsure about the treatment plan, talk to the therapist (and perhaps your child's physician) about your concerns. Or ask for the records and get a second opinion.

After your meeting, you are ready to continue to the next step—finding the right help for your child.

finding the right help

There are three treatment options for depression—talk therapy (psychotherapy), medication or a combination of the two. Different kinds of mental health professionals specialize in these different treatments.

- *Psychiatrists* prescribe and monitor medication. Many psychiatrists only prescribe and monitor medication; they do not practice talk therapy—but some do both.
- *Psychologists, social workers and counselors* practice talk therapy, and often specialize in one particular type of therapy. They are not physicians and therefore they cannot prescribe or monitor medication.

The term "psychotherapist" or "therapist" is not a legal term; rather it's a term we apply broadly to someone who does psychotherapy. Psychiatrists, psychologists, social workers and counselors have specific education, training and state licensing in their fields—it's best to make sure your child's therapist is one of these professionals.

Most states have an on-line option to check whether your therapist is licensed.

Since different kinds of therapists do different things, it can be confusing to find the right person to help your child. To add to the confusion, the mental health community is fragmented—most therapists have private practices, which sometimes makes finding them difficult.

So, given all of this, how do you find the right person?

The treatment plan should tell you what kind of therapist your child needs—it's a good starting point to begin to assemble a list of people who may be right for your child.

We have more information about the different kinds of therapists and therapies in SECTION TWO.

As with the assessment process, you will probably find your child's therapist through referrals. You can begin by asking your child's physician for her recommendations—and once again perhaps she can make a phone call to open the door for you. The person who did the initial assessment may have some names too—in fact, she may become your child's therapist, certainly a convenient option if the personality fit is right.

Networking in your community is also a good way to find names of therapists, and can be an especially good way to find out which therapists are well regarded, and which are not. **In fact, parents who have been through similar circumstances may be your best sources.**

Schools frequently make referrals and can be an excellent source of names. Local mental health social service agencies, hospitals and clinics can be a good source too. Hospitals can be particularly useful if your child suffers from disorders like eating disorders.

Some children may be sufficiently debilitated to require special treatment—hospitalization, a day program they attend instead of school, or a residential therapeutic setting. If your child's pediatrician, therapist or school recommends any of these alternatives, or if you choose to seek any of these because of your concern about your child, you can begin by talking to these professionals to help you make the right decision for your child.

You can also contact the National Association of Therapeutic Schools and Programs (*www.natsap.org*) to find a therapeutic school, or hire an educational consultant who specializes in therapeutic schools. The Independent Educational Consultant Association (*www.iecaonline. com*) is a resource to help you find a consultant in your area.

If your child needs to see more than one therapist—both a psychiatrist to prescribe medication and a talk therapist—finding one may help you find the other. Psychiatrists and talk therapists work regularly with one another and may have a good recommendation for the other half of the team.

At this point, you may be wondering about treatment. Is it safe? Is it effective? There is a lot of controversy today about these two questions. Mental disorders, by their very nature, are difficult to study and therefore different studies have reached different conclusions over the years.

Most mental health professionals, and the American Psychological Association, in its 2006 *Report of the Working Group on Psychotropic Medications for Children and Adolescents*, recommend a conservative approach for treating children and teenagers who have depression—psychotherapy first, with regular monitoring, followed by carefully controlled medication (usually one of the SSRI antidepressants) together with the psychotherapy if the psychotherapy alone is not effective.

If, however, your child is having significant difficulty with daily functioning, has particularly peculiar thinking or behavior, is focused on death, has attempted suicide, or is engaging in self-injury like cutting, it may be best to begin with medication and psychotherapy together.

If the situation is extremely dire— if your child is an immediate threat to himself or others or if he is hearing voices or seeing things that aren't there, you may need to consider hospitalization.

As we mentioned before, the Internet can also be of help. See page 8 for a list of websites that may be helpful.

A list of five to ten names should be sufficient to get you started with the process of finding the right therapist for your child. Why so many? Often therapists are not currently taking new patients (though if you call back in a week or two, their practice may be open) and some therapists, though a good fit for one child, may not be the right person for your child. If a therapist is not taking new patients, ask her for a recommendation.

INTERVIEWING THERAPISTS

Once you have compiled your list, call each person to see whether she is available and willing to treat your child and whether you think she would be a good therapist for your child. You might have to call a few times; many therapists do their own scheduling and are hard to reach. If you think the person is potentially a good fit for your child, set up an interview with her. You will probably want to limit the number of therapists you interview to three or four—this will probably be sufficient for you to find someone who will work well with your child.

At the interview, tell the therapist about your child—age, gender, the reasons (i.e., the moods, behaviors and physical symptoms) that led you to seek help, and the results of your child's mental health assessment. Refer to your journal as a source of information.

Ask the therapist about her practice and her philosophy towards therapy. Here are some questions you can ask during the interview:

[ ] How long have you been practicing therapy?
[ ] What kind of therapy do you practice? Is it in line with my child's diagnosis and treatment plan?
[ ] Do you have special training in, or particular experience with, any particular disorder?
[ ] Do you have special training to treat children and/or teenagers?
[ ] Do you work regularly with my child's age group? Gender?
[ ] Do you feel comfortable treating my child, based on his diagnosis, treatment plan, age and gender?
[ ] How often would you see my child?
[ ] Can my child contact you if he needs to talk about an issue in between sessions? How?
[ ] How do you know whether the therapy is working?
[ ] How can my child tell whether the therapy is working?
[ ] Do you set goals with your patients?
[ ] How do you work with families? Do you generally recommend family therapy?
[ ] Will you meet with me regularly to talk about my child's progress? How frequently? How openly can you discuss what goes on in therapy with me?
[ ] How can I contact you to let you know if something is happening at home or school?
[ ] How can I tell whether the therapy is working?
[ ] Have you ever had a patient who was not a good fit, or whose therapy was not working? How did you handle that situation?
[ ] How would you work with other professionals in my child's life—my child's physician, another therapist, school personnel?
[ ] How do you handle emergency situations?
[ ] How do we know when it's time to end therapy?

Involve your child in this final selection process if you think it's appropriate. Children and teenagers, not surprisingly, often resist the idea of therapy. You may get more buy-in from them if you include them.

Your child's relationship with his therapist is a key to successful therapy. The right personality fit is important.

Some children, like some adults, work better with therapists who are more touchy/feely and some work better with therapists who are more pragmatic or business-like in their approach. Take your child's personality into account when you are interviewing therapists and ask yourself, *"Do I think this therapist will be a good fit for my child?"*

If your child has more than one disorder—depression and an eating disorder, for example—ask the therapist if she has experience with both conditions.

If your child is young, it's important to find someone who works with your child's age group. The younger the child, the greater the difficulty he will have verbalizing his feelings. Special types of therapy may need to be considered. Play, movement or art therapy, for example, might be particularly useful ways for a young child to express his feelings.

Older children and teenagers are likely to need help with their relationships. Relationships with family members are often troublesome. And friendships, which are particularly important to them and so frequently impaired as a result of depression, may be stressors that are contributing to the depression.

If the therapist—psychiatrist—is going to prescribe medication for your child, ask her about her general philosophy on the use of medication to treat depression in children and teenagers. Some psychiatrists are less committed to talk therapy in addition to medication to treat depression—however, **talk therapy should be part of the treatment plan**.

If the therapist—psychiatrist—is going to prescribe medication for your child, make sure you ask how often and which tests or assessments she will use to assess both the effectiveness and side effects of the medication. Of course, it goes without saying that frequent and in-depth monitoring is very important. Some of these medications require regular blood tests to monitor toxicity.

Once you have selected your child's therapist, it's time to begin therapy.

getting treatment

It's not always easy to get your child to go to therapy. We all want to feel that we're normal and there is a considerable amount of stigma in our society about therapy. Don't be surprised if your child thinks he doesn't need therapy, or if he resists going. Explain to your child that going to therapy is not a punishment; it's a chance for him get support through a difficult time and to learn coping strategies that he will use for the rest of his life. Try to keep an upbeat, but firm, stance on the issue.

Your child might be fearful or anxious about going to therapy. This, too, is normal. Acknowledging that you know it's a scary thing for your child might be just what he needs to help him overcome that initial, and understandable, fear.

> Often the biggest barrier to getting your child to go to therapy is denial—it's normal for children, and adults, to deny there is a problem, or deny that they need treatment to help solve the problem.

Watch for moments of opportunity to tap into—moments when your child is vulnerable, when your child knows he needs help, and may be willing to reach out for it. Even if your child is in some degree of self-denial about his depression, such moments exist and they can be breakthrough moments.

TELL YOUR CHILD: "YOU DESERVE TO FEEL BETTER."

If your child is tearful day after day or is withdrawing from activities he previously enjoyed, you may be able to gently broach the subject of therapy. Sometimes just saying, "You deserve to feel better," can open the door to getting him the help he needs.

Keep in mind, too, that therapists are very familiar with the problem of patients who don't want to go to therapy. If you can persuade your child to make two or three visits, that may be enough for the therapist to make a good connection with him. You should be able to tell if it's working—if your child begins to go to therapy sessions more and more willingly, that's a good sign.

Teenagers, in particular, may balk at therapy. They often feel that by right they should be able to determine their own course of action.

If your child refuses to go to therapy, consider going yourself for advance support and to send a healthy message to your child about therapy.

One thing is clear—you can't make someone do something they don't want to do. You can only present the options for them, and tell them why you think it's a good idea to go. *Successful therapy requires that the person in therapy eventually take ownership of his own mental health—and that goes for our children as well as us.* But often, gentle, but firm, prodding can go a long way towards getting a reluctant child or teenager to go to therapy.

STARTING THERAPY

You should also tell the therapist about your child's past health history—other mental disorders, ADHD or learning disorders, allergies, other chronic illnesses and medications, including over-the-counter medications, vitamins and herbal supplements, that your child is taking.

If your child has a history of using tobacco, alcohol or street drugs, the therapist must know that as well.

If your child is refusing or avoiding school, talk to your child's therapist about it. Chapter Four has more information on how to navigate your child's school experience, including a section on school refusal.

Once you have cleared the initial hurdle of going to therapy, it's time to turn your attention to the therapy itself. You, your child and his therapist should have an initial "getting started" meeting. If you didn't do so during the preliminary interview, give the therapist a general history of your child—moods and behavior patterns, a health history, and school performance information.

Think about it as telling your child's story—the more you can paint a picture of your child, his likes and dislikes, his skills and his temperament, the more the therapist will begin to understand your child. Bring your journal to the meeting.

Your child can tell his story from his perspective. Note, however, that the depression itself makes it difficult for people to self-report.

Ask your child's talk therapist about therapy and what to expect.
- [ ] What do the diagnosis and treatment plan mean?
- [ ] What happens during therapy sessions?
- [ ] How frequently will sessions take place?
- [ ] What changes in mood, behavior and physical symptoms will you look for? How soon do you expect them to occur?
- [ ] What changes will my child feel or notice?
- [ ] What changes will we see at home?
- [ ] How can the family help?
- [ ] Are family therapy sessions needed?

[ ] What can the school do to help?

[ ] Will there be "therapy homework?"

[ ] How frequently should we meet to talk about progress?

[ ] How can I contact you to let you know about important issues at home and school?

[ ] How will you work with my child's physician, other therapist and school personnel?

[ ] How can we reach you during an emergency?

[ ] What should we do if a session is missed without excuse?

[ ] How do you know when therapy isn't working? What do you do in those situations?

[ ] How do you know when therapy should be ended?

If your child is going to begin medication as part of his treatment, ask the psychiatrist about the medication she is proposing for your child:

[ ] How does the medication work?

[ ] Which symptoms will the medication alleviate? How long will it be before we see positive results? Do the symptoms disappear all at once or gradually over time?

[ ] How do you know when the medication is working?

[ ] What are the side effects of the medication? What should we do if they occur? Which are serious and which are not? What should we do in the case of a sudden negative side effect?

[ ] How long do you think my child will be on this medication?

[ ] How often will you see my child to monitor the medication?

[ ] What kind of tests will you run to make sure the medication is safe for my child? How often will you do these tests?

[ ] How should the medication be taken? Regularly, at a certain time of day? With or without food, liquids or other medications? Are there any foods or other substances that should be avoided?

[ ] What should we do if a dose is missed?

[ ] What are the potential interactions with other medications, over-the-counter products, tobacco, alcohol, and street drugs?

[ ] Where can I get more information about this medication? Is it approved for use for my child's illness? My child's age group? Can I see the research on the medication?

[ ] What are the long term risks of the medication?

For more information about medication used to treat depression, see SECTION TWO, Chapter Four.

A FEW THIINGS TO NOTE

Teens often self-medicate their depression and anxiety by using alcohol and drugs. Nearly one-third of those with mental disorders also have a substance abuse problem. Untreated depression and anxiety feel less painful when a person is high. However, the feeling is fleeting and the continued use of these substances does not treat the condition and may even make it worse. Be on the lookout for this and be sure to tell your child's therapist if your child is using drugs or alcohol.

If there are others in the family who are also taking medication for a mood disorder and the medication is working well for that person, tell your child's psychiatrist.

Psychotropic: aimed specifically at treating mental disorders.

If your child is taking medication, keep a medication journal. Psychotropic medication takes a while to get right and is frequently adjusted, both the dose and the type—keeping a regular record is a valuable tool to use to determine whether adjustments are needed. Use it to record every time your child takes his medication, the dose taken, and daily reports of feelings, moods, behaviors, physical symptoms, benefits and side effects of the medication. You and your child can both participate in the maintenance of this journal.

If your child is taking medication, monitor when and whether he takes them. It's very common for children and teens to forget, unintentionlly and sometimes very intentionally, to take them. Sudden withdrawal from these medications can be dangerous.

If your child is taking medication, you should make sure that both of his therapists speak to one another regularly. And, make sure your child knows that he can't stop the talk therapy just because he is on medication. Both are important steps towards your child's recovery.

Ask your child's therapist about goal-setting—it's a tool some therapists use. Goal-setting is a process in which the therapist and your child set specific, tangible goals and measurements, or signposts, which they use to assess the progress that's being made in therapy. For example, one goal they might set is a decrease in your child's depressive feelings. The measurements for that goal might be that your child smiles more often at home and joins an extracurricular activity after school. Or they might set a goal of better sleep patterns, and the signposts might be that your child is able to maintain a regular bedtime schedule and wakes feeling refreshed each morning.

A tool you or your child's therapist might wish to use is a journal. Journals can take many forms and be tailored to your child's age, skills and needs—it can be the traditional kind of journal in which your child writes about his thoughts, moods and feelings, it can be a chart of daily activities and progress, including school, or it can also be something as simple as an art journal—drawings done by your child—or a sticker journal, in which your child places stickers to record his moods.

Don't forget about your journal too. Your continuing observations about your child's moods, behaviors and physical symptoms are important.

Journals are an incredibly helpful tool for keeping track of daily changes in moods and other symptoms and for charting things like progress at school and other activities. It's a great way for you, your child and his therapist to be able to understand whether or not he is progressing in a way that is expected, and, if not, to make changes in treatment or daily activities to allow for progress.

In order for your child's therapy to be successful, you and members of your family may need to participate in family therapy. While this can seem like one more thing on your plate, it can be a very useful thing for the child who is suffering from depression, not to mention the family as a whole—sometimes depression is part of a family dynamic and sometimes one member's depression can create a negative family dynamic. It also sends a strong signal to your child that therapy is important and that everyone in the family is working to support one another. Often parents expect their child to be "fixed" by therapy without any changes in family dynamics that may be contributing to a child's depression. Ask your child's therapist if she thinks your child would benefit from family therapy. She can probably help you find a family therapist.

MONITORING THERAPY

Once your child (and perhaps the entire family) is established in therapy, goals are set and journals are being kept, you've made a lot of progress. You should feel good about that. But ... you're not done. At some point, say a month or so into therapy, and then from time to time during the course of your child's therapy, you should check in with your child and meet with your child's therapist to assess whether therapy is going well and whether your child's therapist is a good fit.

These are sometimes tricky questions to ask and there are not always easy answers to them. Therapy is between your child and his therapist. Furthermore, even asking the question begs the next question—what to do if it's not going well. However, these questions need to be asked; you don't want to waste precious time if the therapist isn't a good fit, or if the therapy isn't working.

One way to get a sense of how therapy is going is to sit down with your child and ask him what he thinks.

[ ] How do you feel compared to before you began therapy?
[ ] Do you like your therapist?
[ ] Do you feel respected and comfortable talking to your therapist?
[ ] Do you think she is helping you?
[ ] Do you think you are progressing on your goals?

If you suspect your child is considering suicide, his journal may be a good indication of how serious his depression is.

Depending on your child's age and temperament, you may want to take a look at his journal if he's keeping one. But be sensitive about this issue—an older child may feel you are prying.

Keep in mind a few things when you talk to your child about therapy. The younger the child, the less he may be able to talk about therapy. And, of course, if your child is going to therapy under protest, he may not be the best judge of the effectiveness of the therapy. If your child responds that he hates therapy or it's "stupid" or "pointless," that may not necessarily be the objective case—in fact, it may be difficult for him precisely **because** it's working.

If your child is on medication, ask your child whether he thinks the medication is working, and if he notices any benefits—increased happiness, more interest in daily activities, more energy, better sleep, etc.—or any negative side effects—sleepiness or feeling "wired," appetite changes, changes or swings in mood, especially euphoria or deepening depression, or if he just doesn't feel himself. The medication journal will be a good reference point to use here. Make sure you report any side effects to your child's psychiatrist so she can make adjustments to the medication if need be.

In addition to asking your child about therapy, you should meet with your child's therapist and ask her what her impressions are:

[ ] Do you agree with the initial diagnosis?
[ ] Tell me about your relationship with my child. Do you think you work well together?
[ ] Are you making satisfactory progress towards meeting your goals? Can we review the goals and the progress that's being made?
[ ] How much more time do you think you will need for treatment?
[ ] Are there things we should be doing at home to help?
[ ] Are there things that the school, other therapist or other professionals should be doing?
[ ] Are family sessions recommended?

It's a good idea to tell your child before you meet with his therapist so he doesn't think you are conspiring against him. Include your child in the meeting if you think it's appropriate.

If your child is seeing both a psychiatrist and a talk therapist, ask both therapists how often and effectively they are speaking to one another to coordinate treatment.

A word of caution. Be a little careful about setting up a dynamic where you are calling or meeting with your child's therapist too frequently for a status check. It can be seen by your child, especially if he is older, as interfering. It can also offer your child a handy excuse to avoid taking ownership of his therapy—*if mom or dad is overseeing it, then I don't have to.* Keep in mind that therapy is your child's job, not yours.

Keep in mind when talking to both your child and his therapist(s) that they may be unwilling, or unable, to speak about the details of therapy. Confidentiality is an important part of therapy. Your child needs to know that his therapist will not tell you everything that they are working on in therapy—it needs to be a safe environment for your child to talk about his feelings, which may include feelings about you. On the other hand, the therapist should be forthcoming with you about the success or failure of the therapy, goals, timelines and other more general topics.

Getting medication right can be difficult and often takes trial and error—and patience. If your child is on medication, bring the medication journal along when you meet with the psychiatrist. Tell the psychiatrist about both the benefits—increased happiness, more interest in daily activities, more energy, better sleep, etc.—and negative side effects—sleepiness or feeling "wired," appetitite changes, mood changes or swings, especially euphoria or deepening depression, or if your child just doesn't seem himself—of the medication. Ask how much longer the psychiatrist believes your child will be on the medication. Also ask how she is assessing the effectiveness, and how is she measuring the side effects and safety of the medication.

If you and your child believe the medication is not working as effectively as it should or if the side effects are a nagging problem, talk to the psychiatrist about changing medications or adjusting the dose. It can often take a while to get the medication right and you, your child and his psychiatrist need to be persistent in that effort.

Sometimes you can tell whether your child is progressing in therapy or doing worse by looking at their writing or art at school. If there are projects at school that might give you an insight into his emotional state, ask his teacher if you can see his work.

Again, you need to tread carefully here, especially with older children and teenagers. Looking at their private writing without their permission might provoke their ire, at a price that isn't worth what you got from it.

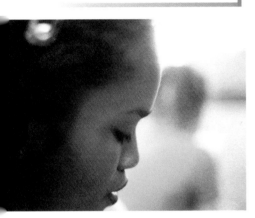

You also are a good touchstone as to whether you think therapy is working well. Review your journal and ask yourself these questions:

[ ] Do I see improvement in my child's mood, behavior and/or physical symptoms?
[ ] Is my child meeting his goals?
[ ] Does my child like his therapist?
[ ] Is the therapist communicating openly and regularly with me?
[ ] Is the therapist accessible to my child?
[ ] Do I think the therapist is helping my child?
[ ] Do I think the therapist is a good fit for my child?

If, after talking to your child and sitting down with his therapist, you are concerned about the progress, or are worried that the fit isn't right between the therapist and your child, talk to the therapist about your concerns. It can be tempting to make a change to another therapist and it's often done and often necessary—but it isn't always a good idea. You may not be seeing significant progress, but this isn't necessarily a sign that therapy isn't working—it may just mean that the hard, sometimes unpleasant, work of therapy is occurring and the benefits are yet to come. "Shopping around" for different therapists when issues get tough, complex or challenging is not helpful to your child.

If, however, in the end, you come to the conclusion that you need to make a change, do so. The relationship between therapist and patient is critical to the success of the therapy, and if you conclude that the relationship just isn't there, or you are unhappy at the progress being made after having given it fair time, it's probably best to begin the process all over again and find another therapist.

This is often easier said than done—it took a lot of effort to find a therapist in the first place, and it is even more difficult to come to the conclusion that the therapist you worked so hard to find just isn't working out. In addition, your child may not want to make a change, or he may take the opportunity to lobby hard for discontinuation of therapy altogether, for the very understandable reason that he has to start all over again. If you find yourself at this place, the list you compiled at the beginning of the process will be a help to you as you travel down this path again.

WORKING TOGETHER

When your child is suffering from depression, one of your jobs is to make sure that the other adults who are a part of your child's daily life—teachers, coaches, tutors, etc.—are aware of what's going on to the extent they need to be. Why? If the right people know about your child's illness—not necessarily the details, but at least the gist—then they can provide a support system for him at times during the day when you are not there.

These people should also let you know when they see something of concern. Ask them to notify you if they notice your child is talking or writing about suicide, physical harm to himself or others, giving away his possessions or saying good-bye to friends. These signs need to be immediately communicated to your child's therapist to see if immediate hospitalization is needed.

By keeping in contact with these people, you are in a better position to help your child deal with troublesome events in his life. For example, if your child is having a difficult time at lunchtime with his friends, talking to your child's therapist and the school about the problem may result in some creative strategies; perhaps the school can ask the lunchroom monitor to temporarily "arrange" seating at lunch. Your child and his therapist can then brainstorm strategies that he can use to make lunchtime less difficult to negotiate. Similarly, if your child's teacher or tutor notices a decline in your child's ability to pay attention, she can let you know and you can report this information to your child's therapist.

However, you will want to take your child's privacy into consideration before speaking to these people. As much as we don't like it, stigma is still an issue when it comes to mental disorders, and your goal in taking these people into your family confidence is to provide a safety net for your child, not to embarrass or humiliate him in any way. Perhaps getting permission from your child beforehand will help you decide which adults to speak to and what to say.

Because school is such an important part of your child's day, we have devoted Chapter Four of SECTION ONE to help you with this subject.

INSURANCE

Many health insurance plans require pre-authorization for mental health claims.

Testing and evaluations for your child's mental health assessment and adjustments to your child's school day may be at least partly covered by your health insurance policy.

HIPAA and privacy—Your child's privacy is protected by the Health Insurance Portability and Accountability Act of 1996 (HIPAA). HIPAA denies current and potential employers access to confidential medical records.

Insurance is perhaps one of the more frustrating issues for parents. It's time-consuming and often confusing. Many therapists do not participate in any insurance plan. The American Psychological Association has a terrific summary of insurance related issues available at *www.apa.org/helpcenter*.

Shortly after, or even before, your child begins treatment, you should contact your insurance company to find out coverage limits so that when you need to make treatment decisions, you know which options you will be reimbursed for and which you will not.

One thing we'd like to say about insurance. Many parents at some point during their child's treatment face having to pay out-of-pocket for treatment because their insurance coverage either doesn't cover the treatment, or their coverage has reached its limits. Some parents prefer to pay out of pocket for their child's therapy in order to protect his privacy. If either of these happen to you, we hope you will be able to find a way to continue your child's treatment. Talk to your child's therapist about your financial concerns—many therapists can offer suggestions and will work with you so that your child can continue with his therapy. We believe it's important that your child get the treatment he needs—and we hope you will find a way to continue it.

You now have your child's therapy in hand, and so now we turn to the home—dealing with your child, other family members … and yourself.

talking to your child

Talking to your child about his depression is often a tricky, and ever-changing, task. Being honest and open with your child about his condition and treatment is a good place to begin.

TALK ABOUT THE DEPRESSION

One thing you can do for your child is to let him know that you support him throughout this process. He needs to know that you love him, that you are able to separate out the depression from the "real" person, and that you will always be there when needed. Tell him: "I notice, I care, it's not your fault and I want to help."

As we have said before, your child, like everyone, wants to be "normal," and may deny he has depression. In fact, this is very common. If you keep an open dialogue with your child, over time he may begin to admit that there is a problem and talk to you about it. Reassure him that you know he is in pain—a pain he deserves to be free from.

These conversations can be difficult, but don't avoid the issue—it's the elephant in the room anyway. Talking can bring you together in ways that will surprise you. But also be prepared for your child to be honest with you about his feelings about you, often unflinchingly, and sometimes dead right. Don't take it too personally and listen, really listen, to what your child is telling you. This may be an important part of his therapy, and it's certainly good modeling for him. Someone in the throes of depression is often touchy about others' criticisms and if you can show him that you can take his constructive criticisms of you, he may begin to do the same.

Your child may be teased by his friends or classmates about his depression. This can be extremely hurtful. If it occurs, let your child's therapist know about it.

Talk to your child about it and let him know that you understand how hurtful this is. Remind him that teasing is often a result of fear. You can brainstorm possible solutions with your child—he can just ignore the teasing or talk to the offender about it, for example.

Talking openly to your child might also foster an atmosphere in which your child can talk to you about other problems he might be having—ancillary problems, like problems with friends or academic issues. Often when a child is depressed, friendships become difficult. Some friends, even long-time ones, may distance themselves from your child.

Be honest with your child. Tell your child that you don't know what the answer to his depression is and that you don't know how or when it will all play out. This is the unhappy truth of dealing with mental disorders—they are unpredictable. But making sure that your child knows that together you will deal with whatever the future holds can be immensely reassuring for him. And of course, tell him that while you may not know the details of how his depression will affect him or when he will get better, make sure you tell him that he **will get better,** with treatment, time—and love.

ENCOURAGE GOOD PHYSICAL AND MENTAL HEALTH

Another way you can help your child is by helping them take care of themselves through nutrition, sleep and exercise.

Depression can wreak havoc on a child's appetite. Your child can have very little appetite, can be eating too much, or can be eating the wrong foods. Helping your child understand the connection between eating habits, depression and energy levels is an important lesson in mental health maintenance.

Encourage your child to eat a good diet and, of course, avoid alcohol, tobacco and street drugs. Encourage your child to eat a good breakfast and make sure he leaves the house with a plan for a balanced lunch and and keep healthy snacks on hand.

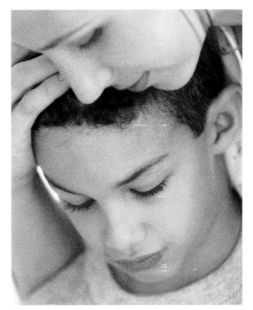

For a child with depression, sleep can be a battle—struggling to fall asleep, stay asleep and getting out of bed in the morning are all common problems for someone suffering from depression. Children and teens should sleep around 9 hours each night. Help your child create a healthy sleep environment—cool, dark, quiet and relaxing. A bedtime ritual may be helpful—taking a shower or bath, reading a book, or listening to quiet music.

It is just as important to help your child understand the activities that should be avoided before bed. In the hour before bedtime, your child should not engage in activities that put the brain in an excited state—things like homework, talking to friends or using a backlit device (cell phones, TV, tablets, video games and computers).

Research indicates that exercise generates "feel good" endorphins that can improve your child's mood. Regular exercise can be as effective as psychotropic medication for cases of mild to moderate depression. As a general rule, your child should strive for 30 minutes a day or 2.5 hours of moderately intensive exercise each week. If your child's depression has made physical activity practically obsolete, start small. Encourage your child to walk or bike to school, take the dog for a walk or go for a run around the neighborhood.

Final thought: Although there are strong mental health benefits to eating right, exercise and good sleep, these practices alone are not a substitute for professional treatment.

SOCIAL LIFE

Your child may separate himself from his friends. It's common for someone who is depressed to have a low level of self-worth. Your child may believe that his friends don't like him. Remind your child that this is the depression speaking—and that he may be perceiving things differently than they really are. And your child's friends may separate themselves from your child. This can be a lonely time for your child. He will need your support.

If your child comes to you, or if you see that friendships are changing, you might want to talk to your child about how he can make things better—even just one loyal friend can be a significant thing for your child. You should also convey this changing environment to your child's therapist so that she can deal with the issue during therapy.

LIFE AT HOME

Your child's relationship with his siblings may also suffer. Siblings often don't understand what is happening, and may be embarrassed, angry, scared or jealous. To make matters more complicated, irritability is a common symptom of depression and siblings are sometimes a target for a depressed child who needs to let off steam (and vice-versa). It can be a tricky situation for you to mediate—but open communication with everyone in the family may help diffuse some of the tension. And family therapy may be an immeasurably useful tool to help everyone in the family deal with these natural tensions.

SCHOOL AND OUTSIDE ACTIVITIES

Another change that you may see is a decline in your child's interest or performance in schoolwork and other activities. He may avoid or even refuse to go to school or particate in outside activities.

Cognitive changes like a drop in grades or the loss of ability to pay attention or concentrate are symptoms of depression and often they are the first signs to appear. In addition, a depressed child feels hopeless and may also be struggling with fatigue—he is likely not too interested in doing homework—or even playing in the back yard after school. You may find yourself spending quite a bit of time monitoring these activities—checking in from time to time with teachers, coaches, etc., and trouble-shooting problems. You may need to be an advocate for your child, especially when times are particularly difficult.

Some children need a break from activities when they are suffering from depression—it may be just too difficult to keep up with schoolwork *and* baseball *and* piano lessons. On the other hand, if your child can stick with some activities that he used to find pleasure in, even just one activity, it may become a valuable part of your child's recovery. Like everything else, it's a balancing act.

But—you will have to choose your battles and, remember, you don't want to win the battle to lose the war. Some activities may need to be dropped and sometimes you need to insist on follow through ... and follow through yourself to make sure your child keeps up with his responsibilities. The more responsibility your child can take for his daily functions, the better. Encourage this and praise it when it occurs.

Your child may need special adjustments at school to help him manage the school day, at least for a while. We have more information on the kinds of help available at school in Chapter Four, including a section on school refusal.

Again, please remember that it will be helpful for your child's recovery if you share all of these at-home issues with your child's therapist so that they can be dealt with in therapy as well as at home.

talking to your family

As if dealing with your suffering child is not enough, you will quickly discover that what your child is feeling has repercussions in your family—both immediate and extended. The child who is suffering may have feelings and questions about his place in the family. Siblings, you, your spouse, extended family—all have different feelings, reactions—and opinions—about what is going on.

**If your child is dealing with depression,
the whole family is dealing with depression.**

Family members will have a myriad of feelings and questions about the condition and behavior of your child. They may be embarrassed, anxious, angry, afraid. They may communicate this to you—they may not.

There can be a genetic component to your child's depression—other family members may be suffering, often with different symptoms. One person may be angry and combative, one may be silent and withdrawn.

Siblings can be especially impacted by the mood disorder of another child in the family. And each sibling, of course, will react in her own way. It is common for siblings to be embarrassed about what's going on—the stigma associated with depression is significant. It's also common for siblings to become withdrawn. They may see that their sibling needs help and view their role as being invisible so as not to cause more tension in the family.

It's important to respect your child's right to his privacy about his depression.

Talking to your child before speaking to other family members will help give you an idea what information your child feels comfortable sharing with other family members, and what information he would prefer to keep private.

Siblings are also often angry or jealous; they are not getting the attention they are used to. And they may be afraid, wondering if they are the next one in the family to "get" depression. If you explain to them what's going on, and help them address their feelings or vent to you about their worry or frustrations, you may be able to help them move to a more positive stance, become more sensitive to the suffering and pain of depression, and even to help support their suffering sibling.

To the extent you are honest and reassuring with all the members of your family about what's going on, you will serve the entire family well—they will see your modeling and may begin to adopt it themselves. If you treat this in a matter of fact and honest way and not a black mark on your child or a permanent personality trait, the rest of the family hopefully will begin to treat it in a similar manner.

But know that this is a process, not a one-time conversation. Remember that your child's siblings are children themselves—all the intellectual conversation in the world may not help them understand that it's the depression talking and not their brother the next time he shouts at them for no good reason or once again gets a bye from you on dishwashing duty.

Try to maintain normal family activities. Go to the movies together. Plan an outing. Eating together even a few nights a week can be an important way of keeping the family together.

Don't forget family therapy—it may help you resolve some of the family dynamic issues so that the whole family can find a way to work together in positive ways to support one another.

You may find that certain family members need to seek individual therapy to help them deal with what's going on. This can be very helpful to a family member who may or may not even know what to think, much less how to feel about this disorder that has invaded her life—and it is powerful indeed for the child who is suffering to see that other family members are getting the help they need too.

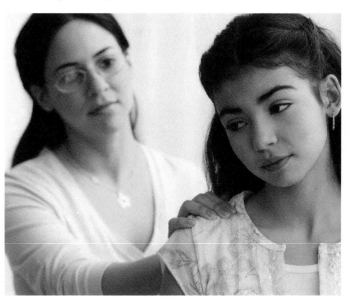

taking care of yourself

At this point, you are probably thinking, *Phew! I need support!*

You probably do—you may need to see a therapist yourself. We have found this to be immensely helpful. A therapist can help in several ways. She can help you deal with your own emotions about what's happening. And she is someone you can bounce ideas off of. Finally, and very importantly, getting yourself into therapy is setting a good example for your child.

**You can't be available to the rest of the family
if you don't take care of yourself.**

One emotion you may be feeling is guilt. Parents often are racked by it—they believe they caused the depression, and they feel totally responsible for it. You may even feel family members or friends judging you. Try to deal with this emotion openly with your therapist.

Another issue that sometimes occurs when a child is suffering from depression is spousal relationships. Sometimes spouses blame one another, sometimes one spouse doesn't believe there is a problem, sometimes spouses disagree over what to do. All of these things are pretty common occurrences. We don't have an easy answer to these issues. Try to talk through your disagreements with an open heart and an open mind. Remember, your spouse knows your child as well as you do and may have a perspective you've never even considered—and he may even be right!

Try to agree, or at least agree to disagree, on the steps you are taking and, remember too that this is a journey and no one decision will make or break your child's recovery. By working together and supporting your child, and his siblings, you will go a long way to stabilizing the family and helping everyone during a difficult time.

You and your spouse may find it beneficial to join a support group. Much like seeing a therapist, talking to people who are in the same place as you are can help in two ways—they can help you deal with your emotions in a safe and understanding environment and they can help you problem-solve some of the daily issues that are difficult for you to sort through.

These organizations can help you find a support group online or in your area:
- [ ] The National Alliance on Mental Illness (*www.nami.org*)
- [ ] The Depression and Bipolar Support Alliance (*www.dbsalliance.org*).

Don't forget your friends. Or your close family members. You should not feel as if you are going through this alone. Call on people close to you to help you—even if it's making dinner for the family or going for a walk. Talking to a trusted friend may be the best thing you do—it's a wonderful thing to be able to confide your darkest fears and deepest emotions to someone who loves you.

You may be hesitant to talk to others about what's going on, but once you begin letting others in, you may be surprised at how many people have been in a similar situation.

Remember the statistics at the beginning of the book. **You are not alone.**

And, please, give yourself a little room for errors. You won't be a perfect parent. No one is, even during the best of times. You will make mistakes, both with your child and with the rest of the family. As we ourselves tell our children—recognize when you have made an error, apologize to the people involved and move forward—so you get on with the things that need attending to.

Hopefully, you can also find time to exercise, sleep, eat a healthy diet, and go to a movie or do some other favorite fun thing—these can be stress-relieving activities for you and it's important that you take the time to do them. They are also good activities for you to model for your child and the entire family. Remember, you can't be available to the rest of family if you don't take care of yourself.

one final thought

Therapy is a journey.

Recovery won't happen overnight. It will take time—you will have setbacks. Expect this at the outset, and know that if you keep at it, even through the setbacks, you will eventually reap the rewards of your hard work—a recovered child, able to get on with life and having learned an important life lesson—that everyone is confronted with difficult issues during the course of their lives, but that resiliency and hard work can be the key to managing through those difficult times.

talking to the school

It's common for parents to hesitate telling anyone at school what's going on when their child is suffering from depression or any mental disorder. As parents, we want to protect our children. We worry that if we tell someone at school, our child may be treated differently—or looked down upon.

But if you can judiciously talk to school personnel about your child's condition and his needs, you and the school can work together to help your child make the best out of a very important part of his day. You need to make sure the school is a good environment and that it's providing the right services to your child.

Who at the school should know about your child's depression? At the very least, your child's advisor, primary teacher and/or classroom teacher should know what's going on. You should also consider telling your child's favorite teacher—having one adult that your child trusts and can go to during the school day can be an incredibly important safety net. Your child's teachers can be a resource for you too. Ask them to advise you of any behavior or school work that is concerning to them, especially anything that indicates that your child is thinking about harming himself or others.

A few words about medication and school policy. State law stipulates that if your child is on medication with side effects that could occur during the school day, the school must know about it.

If your child needs to take his medication during the school day, the school nurse or a designate must administer it.

Think about contacting the school nurse—she may already have an inkling that there is an issue anyway. Many childhood depressions have physical components to them, like headache or stomachache. If the nurse knows ahead of time what's going on with your child, she is in a better position to help if and when your child comes to her office.

Who are these people? The school psychologist performs assessments and evaluations for children who may need special adjustments to their school day, a topic which is discussed in detail later in this chapter. She also often conducts counseling sessions at school.

Social workers and counselors have many different functions in the school. They sometimes lead counseling sessions at school. They also are often in classrooms, working with teachers on classroom dynamics, and in the cafeteria or on the playground to observe and be available to students. Social workers also help school psychologists with assessments and evaluations.

It's also important to talk to one or more of the school's mental health staff—psychologist, social worker or counselor. These people can help your child with his school-related issues. They may also be able to help your child's teacher understand how to make the classroom experience better for your child.

How and what should you tell the school? The way we most effectively communicate with others is face-to-face, so we suggest you begin there. Ask for a meeting with those people you think should know about your child's disorder. Consider asking the principal to attend the meeting, particularly if your child is very young, or suffering particularly acutely.

FOUR
school

Make sure the school knows the appropriate facts about your child's disorder, treatment he is receiving, your thoughts on the ramifications of the disorder for your child's progress at school and your ideas about any changes or adjustments your child may need at school.

You may also want to share information about any social challenges your child is facing. Who your child is sitting with at lunch and whether or not he has been abandoned by friends are important issues. The school should be sensitive to these problems and their effect on your child's ability to function at school.

Think about giving school personnel permission to speak directly with your child's therapist. You can even ask her to attend the meeting. Most therapists are comfortable working with school personnel. But be sure that you talk to her beforehand about which issues she should, and should not, discuss with the school.

It's a good idea to follow up after the meeting with a letter or an email to make sure everyone is on the same page as to the specifics of the discussion, especially if you have come to any agreements with the school about changes to the school day to help your child.

getting help from the school

Now that you've had initial contact with the school, you will want to consider the resources the school has available for your child. We mentioned before that school psychologists or social workers conduct counseling sessions at school. The goal of these sessions is to focus on issues that affect the learning process or other aspects of your child's school day—they may be a real help to your child.

The goal of counseling sessions at school is to focus on issues that affect your child's learning and functioning at school. It is different from individual therapy done outside the school and shouldn't be seen as an alternative to it.

Group counseling sessions are another option to consider. These sessions are usually organized around a specific topic such as bereavement or divorce, or issues like cutting or eating disorders. Schools often call group therapy sessions by different names—friendship groups, support groups, or social skills groups are all common names. Depending on your child's disorder, one of these groups may be helpful to him.

A school should always notify a parent if their child is enrolled in either group or individual therapy at school.

In addition to counseling sessions at school, if your child is having trouble with the school day in a way that significantly affects his ability to learn or to function at school, you may want to, or the school may want you to, consider adjustments to the school day—commonly referred to in educational jargon as modifications, accommodations or interventions—to help your child.

What, exactly, are these adjustments? In general, they are changes to the school day to help your child overcome the disability that's preventing him from being successful at school. They run the gamut from simple changes—changes you negotiate with your child's teacher like sitting in front of the class to help with his attention—to significant changes that must go through a formal process at school.

Some common informal adjustments you may want to consider are:
- Reduced homework expectations.
- Schedule changes, such as taking harder classes later in the day.
- Sitting in the front of the class to improve attentiveness and concentration.
- Advance notice to the teacher that it's a bad day, so that she can be on the watch in case the situation deteriorates.
- An agreed-upon safe place, such as the nurse's office, for your child to go to when he is feeling out of control—and standing permission for him to excuse himself from class when necessary to go to this place.
- Having your child or his teacher chart his progress at school. It may help you all understand whether any school adjustments or outside therapy are helping.

How can you avail yourself of these adjustments? Well, the simple changes are fairly easily done. They are "informal" agreements that you and the school make together. Very simply, you meet and decide what changes should be made. You can begin this process by requesting a meeting with your child's teacher, school principal and other key staff members. If you come to one of these informal agreements, it's wise to document it in writing. Make sure that everyone, particularly the classroom teacher, has a copy of the agreement so that they can make sure they are following it correctly.

Because these informal adjustments can be implemented immediately, you may want to begin with them. If you can come to an agreement with the school in this manner, it is by far the most expedient way to go, and often offers sufficient changes to the school day to help your child.

It's good to be mindful that these changes are ones negotiated between you and the school. Often schools can make these changes easily, but sometimes, changes you think are easy may not be in the eyes of the teacher or school. Fostering an open dialogue often results in more success than outright demands.

Another, more formal, type of adjustment can be used if your child's disorder limits his ability to learn or engage in other activities at school in a more significant way. But they are still relatively simple changes to the school day—like extended testing time.

It's important to regularly monitor informal and Section 504 adjustments to your child's school day—they are not formally overseen at school and busy school staff can sometimes overlook them. Often even little adjustments, if scrupulously followed, can make a big difference in your child's day.

These adjustments are governed by a federal law, known as Section 504 of The Rehabilitation Act of 1973, or simply Section 504, and are generally referred to as "modifications" and/or "accommodations." Section 504 sets forth specific requirements that must be met—your child must "[1] have a physical or mental impairment that substantially limits one or more major life activities; [2] have a record of such impairment; or [3] be regarded as having such impairment" to qualify for Section 504.

FOUR
school

The final and most formal type of adjustment is available under the Individual with Disabilities Education Act (IDEA). Students receiving services under IDEA are given an Individualized Educational Plan, or IEP, which stipulates the services your child will receive and which is monitored on a regular basis by special education staff. These adjustments are called "interventions" and are available to students who have a disability that falls into one of thirteen specific categories. Serious emotional disturbance is the category that children with mental disorders, including depression, may fall into.

Private schools are not required to provide the services required by either Section 504 or IDEA. If your child is at a private school, you will need to work with the school staff to implement informal adjustments.

IDEA has additional requirements. To qualify for an IEP, your child's disability must:
* adversely affect educational performance, and
* require special education services—a modified curriculum and/or instructional support from special education staff.

You may also hear the acronym RtI, Response to Intervention. It's a relatively new law that governs schools' processes for identifying students who need special services. It should not affect your child's access to services.

Section 504 and IEPs sound a lot alike. What's the difference and what's the practical implication of one versus the other? Very simply, IEPs are more substantive changes than Section 504 changes and they are managed by special education staff, ensuring they are implemented and regularly monitored.

However, the downside of both Section 504 and IEPs is that, unlike informal adjustments, you must go through a formal process to obtain services. This can take some time to do.

Both Section 504 and IDEA require that children be put in the most regular or mainstream setting possible. Section 504 requires a student be educated with their non-disabled peers to the extent possible and IDEA requires a child be accommodated in the "least restrictive environment," or LRE.

THE PROCESS

The first step in the process of getting help either through Section 504 or an IEP is requesting a "referral." This is a request for an "evaluation" to see whether or not your child is eligible for special services. The school then decides whether or not to proceed with the evaluation. They will do so if they believe that the disorder has an "adverse educational effect" on the child. (Remember, this can include non-academic disabilities like depression if they affect the child's ability to learn or function at school.)

LEGAL NOTES: Put your request for a referral and evaluation in writing.

When the school agrees to an evaluation and the parent signs a consent for it, the school has 60 school days to complete the evaluation and hold the eligibility meeting.

What is an evaluation? An evaluation is a variety of tests and a review of your child's performance at school. Depending on his disability, the evaluation may include psychological, cognitive and academic testing, speech, vision and hearing assessments, assessments of the child's learning environment and learning style, reviews of student records, observation of the child in class, behavior rating scales, interviews with parents, and social and health histories of the child.

FOUR
school

Be sure to document what's taking place and keep copies of all correspondence between you and the school.

Evaluations are done by a team of school personnel, typically including the school psychologist, and are done free of charge to the family. If your child has had testing done outside the school—either for his disorder or for a learning disability—give this information to the school so they can consider it during the evaluation.

If you wish to, you can have an evaluation performed by a professional outside of the school at your own expense. The school is obligated to review the evaluation but it does not have to agree with its conclusions and it may decide to conduct an evaluation of its own.

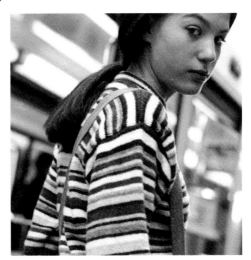

After the evaluation has taken place, a "multi-disciplinary conference" (MDC), which includes parents and school personnel, takes place. An MDC is an "eligibility meeting" to discuss the child's eligibility for services and for which type of services.

If the school agrees that services are needed, an educational plan will be developed. If services are to be provided under IDEA, an IEP will be written that documents the goals and the instructional services and/or modifications to the curriculum to be provided. If services are to be provided under Section 504, a 504 Plan will be written. Make sure you get a copy of whatever plan is developed and read it to be sure it reflects what was agreed upon at the eligibility meeting, or any other meeting, that you attended. You will be asked to sign these documents—if you are unsure about them, tell the school that you would like more time to consider them (and perhaps consult with your child's therapist or others).

Any services agreed to by the school are free of charge to the parent. If the school is not able to provide them, they are obligated to pay for them.

A FINAL WORD

The issues of adjustments to your child's school day are sometimes difficult—as we said before, mental disorders are often hard to diagnose and difficult for some people to accept as real, so it's probably no surprise that people will differ over whether and how to offer adjustments to the school day to accommodate a mental disorder like depression. Because of this, you may find yourself disagreeing with the school over the issue. If you do, both Section 504 and IDEA provide for an impartial hearing process, called a "due process hearing." You can ask for a hearing at any point in the process. Mediation is one possible way of handling the dispute, and attorneys who specialize in special education law can help you with both mediation and a due process hearing.

privacy and school records

What about your child's privacy? When you tell any member of the school community about your child's condition, you can also tell that person who else she may share this information with and who she should not. But keep in mind that this can be a double-edged sword. Your goal is to make sure that the right people at the school know so that your child will be well served—while also protecting your child's privacy to the extent possible. You must balance these two competing needs.

FOUR
school

However, you should know that school policy also dictates who at school will be notified of your child's disorder—ask the school what their policy is and who will be informed as a result of it.

The Family Education Rights and Privacy Act of 1974 (FERPA) is a federal law that protects the privacy of school records, but under the law, faculty and staff can access the student's record if there is a legitimate academic need—so even though the privacy law exists, your child's privacy is not necessarily totally protected.

Furthermore, and understandably, under some circumstances, school personnel are **not** allowed to maintain confidentiality about your child's condition— they are required by law to report instances where they believe a child may be a danger either to himself or to others. Depending on the behavior of the child, that information may be shared within the school building, within the school district, or it may be shared with outside personnel (local law enforcement officials, the state Department of Children and Family Services or medical personnel).

What about school records? There are two types of records that the school creates for each child, both of which follow a child from school to school.

The permanent record is accessible to parents, but no one is allowed to remove information from it.

The first is called the **permanent** record. It contains report cards, attendance information, general information on school performance and a health record—height, weight and the results of screenings for vision and hearing. But it gets a bit muddy here—some schools include information about medication (particularly if the school has been asked to dispense it) or about a specific illness or disorder in the health record portion of the permanent record.

The second type of record is called a **temporary**, or sometimes **confidential**, record. This file contains IEPs and Section 504 Plans, psychological testing results, standardized test data, and all of the health information not contained in the permanent record. This information is available to parents and, unlike the permanent record, it can be excised. School policy and state (the School Records Act) and federal (FERPA) law stipulate the process.

If you wish to see your child's files and/or request that information be removed from the temporary record, ask your child's classroom teacher or advisor who you should contact. If you wish to remove information, be sure to put the request in writing. If the school refuses to remove the information, you have a right to a records hearing under both state and federal law.

Once again, though, if you are considering removing information from the temporary record, be certain to consider all sides of the issue. On the one hand, you want to protect your child's privacy. On the other hand, it's important that your child's schools have the information they need to best meet the needs of your child.

school refusal

It is not uncommon for a child or teen with depression to avoid or refuse to go to school. Inability or reluctance to wake up and get dressed in the morning, frequent visits to the school nurse, skipping class, or frequent complaints of physical pain and sickness like headaches, stomach-aches, nausea, or diarrhea can all be signs of school refusal. Anxiety and defiance may be present as well.

FOUR
school

As a parent, it is hard to know what to do. The behavior can be disruptive to the family and it's heart-wrenching to see your child in pain and unable to manage school. However, the most important step in dealing with school refusal is to understand why your child is having difficulty getting to school. School refusal is often a manifestation of a disorder like depression or anxiety, but it can also be the result of bullying or issues with friends or family members.

If your child is avoiding or refusing to go to school, talk to your child's therapist. She can help develop strategies to help resolve the situation, such as addressing your child's sleeping habits so that he is ready for school in the morning. If it is an issue of bullying, the school should be involved in order to mediate the situation between the bully and your child.

Regardless of the reason for school refusal, it is probably a good idea to get your child's school involved. The school may have ideas about how to help. However, with more people involved, communication is king. Make sure releases are signed so that the school can work with you and your child's therapist seamlessly, resulting in a consistent approach that is supportive and, ultimately, effective.

Everyone's situation is different, and therefore, blanket advice on this topic is not fitting. However, there are a few tips that we have found helpful.

- **Avoid engaging in a power struggle**. When your child is refusing to go to school, try to avoid getting upset. This can escalate the situation and cause both you and your child stress—not a helpful headspace for a child already having trouble going to and/or staying in school.
- **Validate how he must be feeling**. Think about what would be helpful to you if you were in your child's shoes. It would probably feel pretty comforting to know that your mom or dad understands that you are in pain and that getting to school is hard.
- **Reinforce the plan**. Remind your child of the plan in place. If part of the plan is using skills learned in therapy, ask your child's therapist to teach you the skills so you can help. Review those skills with your child each day until he starts to integrate them regularly. Ask your child if it's okay for teachers to be cued in so they can support your child when needed.
- **Establish a safe space**. Often when a child is experiencing emotional difficulty in school, there is a fear of visibly "losing control" in front of his classmates. This may be why he is avoiding school. One way to make the school day feel safer for your child is to ask the school to establish a safe place where he can go to collect himself—a social worker's or nurse's office.

- **Practice patience**. Be firm on the idea of going to school and also understand that overcoming school refusal may take time.
- **Reward and praise improvement**. Make sure to point out the moments when your child is using his skills or making even the smallest steps in the right direction. Remember, when you are depressed, you see failure in everything. Positivity is very powerful.

Chronic school refusal may mean a therapeutic school environment is needed for your child. Talk to your child's school if you believe this step is necessary, as it can sometimes be difficult to get the school's buy-in. The Individuals with Disabilities Education Act (IDEA) requires that a school must provide children with the least restrictive educational environment. For a child exhibiting chronic school refusal, this means that every available school intervention must be exhausted before a school district will fund a therapeutic school placement.

If you have the resources, you may decide to initiate the process on your own. If you decide to do this, you can talk to your child's pediatrician or therapist, who may have some suggestions for you. You can also contact the National Association of Therapeutic Schools and Programs (*www.natsap.org*) to find a school, or hire an educational consultant who specializes in therapeutic schools. The Independent Educational Consultant Association (*www.iecaonline.com*) is a good resource to help you find a consultant in your area.

FOUR
school

definitions and symptoms

What is depression? Depression is officially categorized as a mental disorder—that is, a condition whose symptoms are behavioral or psychological in nature as opposed to physical. Mental disorders are characterized by alterations in mood, thinking and/or behavior. Depression is an alteration of mood; thus it is classified as a mood disorder.

Note the use of the word "disorder" in the definition. This has important implications—it means that we don't "cause" it—and it means that treatment is often necessary for recovery, just as treatment is often necessary to recover from physical illness.

There are many different categories of mental disorders. Other than mood disorders, common mental disorders that affect children and adolescents are:

* anxiety disorders
* conduct disorder
* ADHD (attention deficit-hyperactivity disorder)
* substance-related disorders
* eating disorders
* learning disorders.

Depression in a clinical, or medical, sense has a very specific definition, at least on paper. This medical definition is designed to strike a difference between depression, the mood disorder, and a depressed mood. Everyone feels sad sometimes—that's part of daily living—and teenagers especially feel the angst of growing up.

Major Depressive Disorder (MDD) and Major Depression (MD) are the two terms used by the medical profession for what we commonly call depression.

OFFICIAL DEFINITION OF DEPRESSION

The official definition used to diagnose depression is taken from the *DSM-V* (the American Psychiatric Association's diagnostic manual). Depression, according to the manual, is the presence of at least five of the following symptoms (at least one must be either a depressed mood or loss of interest or pleasure) for at least a two-week period, and representing a change from previous functioning:

- Depressed mood most of the day, nearly every day, as indicated by either subjective report (e.g., feels sad, empty, hopeless) or observation made by others (e.g., appears tearful). *Note: In children and adolescents, can be irritable mood.*
- Markedly diminished interest or pleasure in all, or almost all, activities most of the day, nearly every day (as indicated by either subjective account or observation).
- Significant weight loss when not dieting or weight gain (e.g., a change of more than 5% of body weight in a month), or decrease or increase in appetite nearly every day. Note: In children, consider failure to make expected weight gain.
- Insomnia or hypersomnia nearly every day.
- Psychomotor agitation or retardation nearly every day (observable by others, not merely subjective feelings of restlessness or being slowed down).
- Fatigue or loss of energy nearly every day.
- Feelings of worthlessness or excessive or inappropriate guilt (which may be delusional) nearly every day (not merely self-reproach or guilt about being sick).
- Diminished ability to think or concentrate, or indecisiveness, nearly every day (either by subjective account or as observed by others).
- Recurrent thoughts of death (not just fear of dying), recurrent suicidal ideation without a specific plan, or a suicide attempt or a specific plan for committing suicide.

The symptoms cause clinically significant distress or impairment in social, occupational or other important areas of functioning. The episode is not attributable to the direct physiological effects of a substance or to another medical condition.

Meeting these criteria doesn't necessarily mean a person has depression. Certain medical conditions, like thyroid disease, adrenal gland disease and diabetes, can cause many of the same symptoms. Depressive symptoms can also be a result of bereavement, alcohol abuse, street drugs or the side effects of prescription medications. All of these possibilities need to be ruled out by your child's physician or therapist before a diagnosis of depression is made.

Frequent and persistent thoughts of death or suicide, or suicide attempts, are always categorized as severe depression and need immediate attention and treatment.

There are varying degrees of depression: mild, moderate and severe. As you might expect, in cases of mild depression, the sufferer has sufficient symptoms for a diagnosis, but the symptoms interfere only minimally with daily life. At the opposite end of the spectrum is severe depression, in which an individual is essentially incapacitated—unable to attend school or work, even perhaps unable to get out of bed or take care of himself.

There are known risk factors for depression. These include a family history of depression or suicide, family dysfunction, prenatal damage from alcohol abuse, street drugs, medication, tobacco or other trauma, low birth weight, poverty, abuse, neglect and multiple, frequent life stressors. Children who are the victims of bullying and children who identify as LGBTQ (lesbian, gay, bi-sexual, transgender or queer) are at a higher risk for depression.

It's important to note that these are risk factors, not definitive predictors. In other words, these conditions put a person at a higher risk for depression, but they do not cause the disorder and their presence does not necessarily mean that the disorder will manifest itself. In fact, researchers believe that some combination of genetic and environmental factors are responsible for triggering mental disorders like depression.

In addition to the symptoms outlined in the *DSM-V*, children and adolescents who have depression frequently exhibit physical symptoms like headaches, stomachaches and other aches and pains and they may show more socially-isolating symptoms like neglect of appearance and hygiene. Cognitive symptoms like a drop in grades or difficulty making decisions or paying attention are often the first to appear.

Remember, the symptoms must be sustained over a period of weeks or months in order for there to be a diagnosis of depression.

ONE
definitions
and symptoms

The symptoms of depression vary with age. A depressed infant may show too little or too much crying, lethargy, a sad or deadpan expression, little motor activity, feeding or sleeping problems, lack of attention, lack of curiosity and a failure to grow and thrive.

Symptoms in early elementary school-aged children (ages 6 to 8) may include, in addition to the above general symptoms, poor performance in school, separation anxiety, phobias, accident-proneness and attention-seeking behavior.

It's important to note that young children are generally not able to verbalize their feelings—their depression may manifest itself with anxiety, negative behavior patterns and physical complaints.

Older elementary-schoolers and middle-schoolers (ages 9 to 12) may say they feel "stupid" or use other self-deprecating language. They may have low self-esteem and may feel unloved, and unlovable. They may be reluctant to go to school. More severe symptoms, like thoughts of suicide, sometimes appear at these ages.

Adolescents may talk about the future pessimistically. Running away, cutting or other self-injury, extreme aggressiveness, inattention to appearance, excessive risk-taking behavior and refusal to go to school are also symptoms.

Depressed children and adolescents are often irritable—and their irritability sometimes leads to aggressive behavior.

Anxiety is a frequent precursor to depression in children and adolescents. In fact, depression is frequently seen in tandem with other mental disorders. The 1999 *Mental Health: A Report of the Surgeon General* reports that two-thirds of those who suffer from depression also suffer

from another mental disorder and that, except for substance-related disorder, the depression is secondary (in other words, it arises after, and perhaps in response to, the other disorder).

The most frequent co-occurring disorders are dysthymia, also called persistent depressive disorder (defined later in this chapter), anxiety disorders, conduct disorder, substance-related disorders, ADHD (attention deficit-hyperactivity disorder) and learning disorders.

Research tells us that between 15 and 20% of youth will suffer from at least one depressive episode before they reach adulthood. Before age 15, depression occurs about as frequently in boys as girls; after age 15, twice as many girls suffer from it. Girls are more likely than boys to attempt suicide, but attempts by boys more frequently result in death.

Depression is thought of more and more as a condition to be managed, rather than cured.

Most depressive episodes last between seven and nine months. Most people who suffer from depression will experience a relapse, especially if the first episode is early in life. Between 20% and 40% of children and adolescents will relapse within two years of a first episode, and 70% will relapse by adulthood. The relapses are usually more severe than the previous episodes.

Research on the most effective treatments for depression is ongoing. You can stay abreast of it by talking to your child's therapist and doing your own research on the Internet.

These websites have information about research currently being conducted:
- *bbrfoundation.org*
- *Clinicaltrials.gov*
- *Medlineplus.gov*
- *Nimh.nih.gov*
- *Psychcentral.com*
- *Pdrhealth.com*

However, the news is not all bad. There is research evidence that supports relieving the symptoms of depression with treatment. A well-established base of clinical data (from real-life, as opposed to research, settings) supports the benefits of treatment, too.

Most mental health professionals today and the American Psychological Association, in its 2006 *Report of the Working Group on Psychotropic Medications for Children and Adolescents,* who reviewed all of the then-available literature, recommend a conservative approach for treating children and adolescents suffering from depression—psychotherapy first, with regular monitoring, followed by carefully controlled medication (typically one of the SSRI antidepressants) together with the psychotherapy if the psychotherapy alone is not effective. If a child is having a significant amount of trouble with daily functioning, has particularly peculiar thinking or behavior, is focused on death, has attempted suicide or is engaging in self-injurious behavior like cutting, it may be appropriate to begin with medication and psychotherapy as a combination treatment. If the situation is extremely dire—a child is an immediate threat to himself or others or if he is hearing voices or seeing things that aren't there—hospitalization may be necessary.

ONE
definitions
and symptoms

We believe that it's important for you to get help for your child if he is suffering from depression. Why? An individual with depression is at an increased risk for suicide. Ditto for substance abuse. And, as we mentioned before, 70% of children and adolescents who have a depressive episode suffer from a recurrence by adulthood.

Factors that predict recurrence include the age of onset (earlier being worse), the severity and duration of the preceding episode, the number of previous episodes, the presence of other mental disorders and the presence of life stressors. Note in particular two of these factors—duration and severity; if treatment can mitigate them, then the hope is that it can reduce the occurrence and/or severity of future episodes.

For a child or adolescent suffering from depression, seven, eight or nine months is a very long time—a time when he could be getting on with the business of being a child or teenager—learning, cementing relationships and participating in the variety of activities that will help him recognize and realize his potential.

Research on the plasticity of the brain reinforces the notion that treatment is better than no treatment. The scientists who are looking at this issue hypothesize that depression somehow suppresses the brain's ability to make new brain cells—a process called neurogenesis—and that treatment corrects this, thereby promoting recovery. The brain literally rewires, and heals, itself.

OTHER MOOD DISORDERS

There are a few other mood disorders we would like to spend a little time talking about. The first is dysthymia. Dysthymia (pronounced *dis-THIGH-mee-ah*), or Dysthymic Disorder (also called Persisent Depressive Disorder) is a mood disorder similar to mild depression, but is characterized by the fact that it lasts for at least a year, and often several years. The average duration for children and adolescents is four years. It's a tough mood disorder—its symptoms are generally not enough to interfere significantly with a child's daily life, but they can include socially-isolating symptoms like chronic pessimism and poor social skills. And while it may not interfere with daily life, dysthymia's long duration can mean it affects normal development as much and sometimes more than depression might. Furthermore, dysthymia often persists for so long that parents and even the child may come to believe it's just a matter of temperament—that this is the normal state of being for this child. Dysthymia puts a child at increased risk for depression.

Bipolar disorder (sometimes referred to as manic-depressive disorder) is a complex, difficult to diagnose mood disorder. Very generally, it is characterized by cycling moods: depression followed by mania, followed by depression. The first manifestation is usually a depressive state, with the same characteristics as those of depression. The manic states are ones of persistent euphoric, expansive or irritable moods and may include inflated self-esteem, grandiosity, decreased need for sleep, talking too much or speaking too rapidly, racing or a continuous stream of thoughts, agitation, distractibility, and excessive involvement in pleasurable activities. The mania can occur just after a depressive state, months or even years afterwards, or it can occur simultaneously with the depressive state.

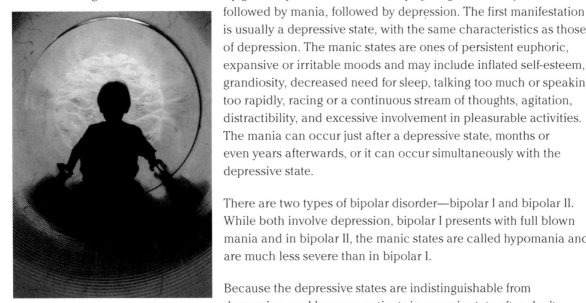

ONE
definitions
and symptoms

There are two types of bipolar disorder—bipolar I and bipolar II. While both involve depression, bipolar I presents with full blown mania and in bipolar II, the manic states are called hypomania and are much less severe than in bipolar I.

Because the depressive states are indistinguishable from depression, and because patients in a manic state often don't recognize that they are ill or they refuse treatment, mental health professionals can have a difficult time diagnosing, much less treating, bipolar disorder. It often takes several cycles before an accurate diagnosis is made. Furthermore, bipolar disorder, because so many of its symptoms mimic ADHD (attention deficit-hyperactivity disorder), is often misdiagnosed as that, particularly in younger children (and, conversely, sometimes ADHD is misdiagnosed as bipolar disorder).

Many children and adolescents with bipolar disorder have other mental disorders as well—most commonly ADHD, conduct disorder, anxiety disorders and, particularly during adolescence, substance-related disorders.

Some who suffer from bipolar disorder have a particularly intense form of the disease—rapid cycling bipolar disorder—in which sufferers can have several cycles in even one day. Children and adolescents can also suffer from mixed-state bipolar disorder, in which the depressive and manic episodes are present at the same time.

A milder form of bipolar disorder is called cyclothymia (*sigh-clo-THIGH-mee-ah*) or Cyclothymic Disorder. Cyclothymic children are kids we might call "moody" or "high-strung." They have unstable moods—cycling rapidly through periods of despair, then joy, followed by discouragement, self-confidence, and then discouragement once again, but never exhibiting the full-blown episodes of mania or depression seen in bipolar cases.

This is but a short summary of mood disorders. If your child is suffering from one of these disorders, or any mental disorder, you may want to do more research on the Internet. Here are some websites which may be helpful:

- The American Psychological Association (*www.apa.org*)
- Anxiety and Depression Association of America (*www.adaa.org*)
- Brain and Behavior Research Foundation (*www.bbrfoundation.org*).
- Children and Adults with Attention Deficit-Hyperactivity Disorder (*www.chadd.org*)
- The Depression and Bipolar Support Alliance (*www.dbsalliance.org*)
- *Healthfinder.gov*
- International OCD Foundation (*www.iocdf.org*)
- *Mayoclinic.org*
- *Medlineplus.gov*
- Mental Health America (*www.mentalhealthamerica.net*)
- The National Alliance on Mental Illness (*www.nami.org*)
- The National Institute of Mental Health (*www.nimh.nih.gov*)
- National Eating Disorders Association (*www.nationaleatingdisorders.org*)
- *Pdrhealth.com*
- *Psychcentral.com*

therapists

During your child's treatment for his depression, he will work with one or more therapists—a psychiatrist, psychologist, social worker or counselor—who either practices talk therapy (psychotherapy) or prescribes medication. **Who are these people and what is their training and education?**

PSYCHIATRISTS

Psychiatrists are physicians who specialize in mental disorders. They have completed both medical school and an additional four-year residency in psychiatry. Some psychiatrists also complete a further specialty in child and adolescent psychiatry.

In addition to their formal education, most psychiatrists become certified by The American Board of Psychiatry and Neurology (*www.abpn.com*). Child and adolescent psychiatrists may be additionally certified in their specialty. Psychiatrists must be licensed by the state in which they practice.

AN IMPORTANT NOTE ABOUT HOSPITALIZATION AND THERAPISTS. Your child's therapist will not be able to see your child while he is in the hospital unless she is a staff member at the hospital or unless the attending physician at the hospital writes an order to permit it.

If your child requires hospitalization, you may want to consider taking him to the hospital where his therapist is on staff; otherwise, make sure an order is written so that she can see your child and participate in his care. Continuity of care and planning for a smooth transition home is important.

Because of their extensive training, psychiatrists have experienced an extremely broad spectrum of conditions—this can be important in the assessment and diagnosis process.

If your child needs medication for his depression, he will need to see a psychiatrist—they are the only mental health professionals who can prescribe medication. In fact, many psychiatrists do only this, and will likely be part of a team that you assemble for your child, as opposed to one therapist who will provide both the medication and talk therapy parts of the treatment.

Psychiatrists generally work in private practice, university-affiliated clinics and at hospitals.

PSYCHOLOGISTS, SOCIAL WORKERS AND COUNSELORS

Psychologists. There are different kinds of psychologists—those who practice therapy are called clinical psychologists. (Experimental, cognitive and social psychologists focus on research, developmental psychologists work with very young children who are not developing normally and school psychologists focus on testing and evaluation for learning disorders.)

Clinical psychologists hold a degree in psychology—at least a master's degree and usually a Ph.D. (doctor of philosophy) or a Psy.D. (doctor of psychology). In addition, clinical psychologists must have completed some period of time, usually two years, of supervised clinical practice and must be licensed by the state in which they practice. Clinical psychologists can become certified by the American Board of Professional Psychology (*www.abpp.org*) and some obtain additional certification in specialties such as clinical psychology, child and adolescent psychology, neuropsychology and cognitive and behavioral psychology.

It's important once again to note that there is a difference between clinical psychologists, who practice individual therapy, and school psychologists, whose expertise is in school testing and evaluations. We emphasize this distinction because people sometimes confuse the two. If your child is seeing the psychologist at his school, those sessions are specifically aimed at issues related to learning and the school environment and are not a substitute for the therapy needed to treat your child.

Social workers. Like clinical psychologists, clinical social workers practice talk therapy—but their university degree is in social work. Most clinical social workers have at least a master's degree (M.S.W.) and sometimes they have a doctorate (D.S.W. or Ph.D.). These degrees require supervised clinical work and, to practice, social workers must be licensed by the state in which they work, signified by the letters L.C.S.W. Social workers can also become certified by the National Association of Social Workers (*www.socialworkers.org*).

Counselors. Counselors also provide therapy, often in community health center and mental health agencies. Counselors have a master's degree in counseling (M.A.C.) and, like psychologists and social workers, have completed supervised clinical work. They must be licensed by the state in which they work, signified by the letter L.P.C., L.M.H.C., L.C.P.C. or L.P.C.C. depending on the state They can also become certified by the National Board for Certified Counselors (*www.nbcc.org*).

As we said before, the role of the psychologist, social worker or counselor is talk therapy. What's the difference between these professionals? Mostly their education. A psychologist's education is in the broad field of psychology—the study of human behavior. A social worker or counselor focuses more on the interactions of individuals and groups. Having said that, the distinction may not be particularly useful in choosing one over the other when you are selecting your child's therapist—all are required to spend time in supervised clinical settings in order to be certified and licensed to practice therapy. In the end, it's really most important to choose someone who:

Although they cannot prescribe and monitor medication, many psychologists, social workers and counselors work with clients who take medication for their depression. Your child's psychologist, social worker or counselor may be a good sounding board for you to determine whether or not his medication is working well, and whether there are other alternatives.

- has a formal education and the proper training to be a qualified therapist
- has a broad range of experience
- works well with your child.

In addition, because different therapists practice different types of therapies (which are discussed in the next chapter), it's important that you know which type of therapy your child's therapist practices—and that this type of therapy meets the needs of your child.

One important note of difference between a clinical psychologist, social worker or counselor is that clinical psychologists, like psychiatrists, generally have more expertise in assessment than do social workers or counselors. You may want to consider this difference when choosing someone to do your child's initial mental health assessment.

Psychologists, social workers and counselors generally work as solo practitioners in private practice, or with other therapists in a group practice. They can also be found at local social service agencies. Very often these agencies are a gateway for people who need help. Hospitals also often have psychologists, social workers and counselors as part of their mental health staff, especially in their clinics. Police departments and schools also often employ counselors, social workers and psychologists (however, that they may not be trained for clinical practice) and these people are often the first people who see children and adolescents who are in crisis—they often have a wealth of information about local services.

OTHER KINDS OF THERAPISTS OR COUNSELORS

There are other kinds of therapists or counselors you may be referred to during the course of your child's treatment: art therapists, marriage and family therapists and addiction counselors are among the list.

Art therapists, as the name implies, use art as an expression of emotion and may be particularly useful for younger children or those who have a difficult time verbalizing their thoughts and feelings.

A marriage and family therapist (M.F.T. or L.M.F.T.) may also be appropriate for your child or family. Marriage and family therapists specialize in family dynamics. They treat both individuals and families by focusing on family relationships and the issues that are causing discord in the family.

Religious institutions often have pastoral counselors, and schools often employ school counselors.

Addiction counselors help people with their addiction.

Many of these therapists and counselors have attended an accredited program to train them in their practice and many are licensed by the state. However, some are not. Hopefully, the person who referred you to a particular therapist or counselor knows the background and credentials of the person she referred you to, but you should also check credentials and references.

talk therapy

Has anyone on the planet not heard of Freud and his impact on how we see ourselves and others? It's really quite profound, and we have much to thank Freud for. However, psychotherapy has changed a lot in the past few decades—it is no longer the familiar "Freudian" psychoanalysis that has Woody Allen lying on the couch in the therapist's office talking about his mother.

The advent of psychotropic drugs in the 1970s was a watershed event. These drugs changed the way we looked at mental disorders—the very fact that they worked forced us to consider that mental disorders are at least partly biologically based and not solely a result of past experiences. Because of this, therapists began to explore new kinds of talk therapies— therapies aimed more at helping patients change their behaviors than analyzing past experiences and memories. Their focus was less on the "why," but rather on helping patients in a very practical way to change their belief systems and behaviors; they are more rooted in the present than the past.

THREE
talk therapy

Many therapies today blend the two viewpoints, borrowing some techniques from the newer "behavior modification" trends and some from the more traditional "analysis" therapies. Therapy for children and adolescents in particular tends to be focused on the "behavior modification" end of the spectrum—children have less of a past to analyze.

We can summarize (and it is a summary indeed) the kinds of therapy that are most commonly practiced today into three basic types: psychodynamic psychotherapy, behavioral therapies and interpersonal therapy.

COMMON KINDS OF THERAPY

Psychodynamic psychotherapy. Psychodynamic psychotherapy (also called dynamic psychotherapy, psychoanalytic psychotherapy, insight-oriented psychotherapy or exploratory psychotherapy) is perhaps closest to what we think of as traditional Freudian therapy. Psychodynamic psychotherapy aims at helping patients discover the unconscious source of their mental disorder. It often focuses on childhood experiences and repressed memories—discovering the root of the problem allows the patient to "let go" of his negative feelings and behaviors. Psychodynamic psychotherapy is not the mainstay therapy today, but some therapists use it occasionally during therapy sessions when they see the need for deeper analysis of motives and behaviors.

Behavioral therapies. Behavioral therapies are on the other end of the continuum from psychodynamic psychotherapy. They are time-limited, practical, problem-focused approachs in which the patient literally works to retrain his thinking.

The most commonly practiced, and studied, behavioral therapy is **cognitive behavioral therapy** (**CBT**). It is aimed at helping the patient understand that his distorted beliefs about himself and the world lead to negative feelings and then to counterproductive behaviors, which cycle back to reinforce his distorted belief system. If he can break one link in the chain, by learning coping skills to counteract the distorted beliefs, the cycle is broken, the distorted beliefs are corrected and the symptoms are reduced in a process called "cognitive restructuring."

Another behavioral therapy that is increasingly used is **dialectical behavior therapy** (**DBT**). DBT is similar to CBT in that it works towards cognitive restructuring but adds, among other things, a component of mindful awareness to the treatment plan.

Interpersonal therapy. Interpersonal therapy (IPT) focuses on improving the patient's interactions with others. Like CBT and DBT, there is less focus on the "why" of behaviors or on the past; rather the focus is on the now and on practical strategies for helping the patient problem-solve and improve his relationships, and thereby feel better about himself. Because of its emphasis on relationships, IPT (in a form specifically designed for adolescents called IPT-A, or Interpersonal Therapy for Adolescents) is sometimes used for adolescents, when peer and parent relationships are so very important.

CBT and IPT-A are the only two forms of talk therapy that have been systematically studied to treat depression in adolescents. These studies generally (though not always) confirm the benefits of both treatments, at least for the short term.

Even though talk therapies like CBT, DBT and IPT are time-limited, repeated courses may be needed to address relapses.

CBT, DBT and IPT/IPT-A have not been well studied in children. In fact, some therapists believe that cognitive approaches are more difficult for this age group because children are not ready for these higher-level thinking activities.

OTHER KINDS OF THERAPY

There are other kinds of therapies—non-directive supportive therapy, narrative therapy, animal therapy, eye movement desensensitization and reprocessing (EMDR), etc.—that you may run across, but none have been well studied. Many websites explain these newer therapies if you are considering them for your child.

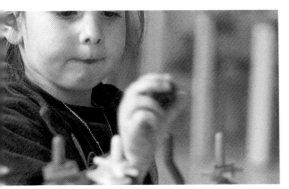

There are also therapeutic techniques that your child's therapist may use from time to time, or even most of the time, during therapy sessions—play, movement and art therapy are three of them. These techniques can help your child's therapist understand your child's emotional state in non-verbal ways—which may be particularly appropriate for younger children or children and adolescents who have a difficult time verbalizing their thoughts and feelings.

THREE
talk therapy

Psychoeducation is a word you might hear about, too. It is being used more and more as an adjunct to any treatment of depression. Psychoeducation is simply educating the patient and his family about depression. From a common sense standpoint, psychoeducation seems like a good idea. The more we can learn about a mood disorder, the more we can understand and relate to the family member who is suffering—and that can only be a good thing. It should be a normal part of all therapy.

Group and Family Therapies. In addition to the individual therapies above, group therapy is a common form of therapy practiced today, particularly when a patient's issues are part of the dynamics of the family or a peer group. There are two basic types of group therapy—family therapy and peer-to-peer group therapy.

If your child is in individual therapy, you, other family members and/or your child may be asked to attend family therapy sessions. The goal of family therapy is to change the dynamics in a family—sometimes family dynamics can contribute to one member's depression and sometimes one member's depression can set in motion a family dynamic that impacts everyone in a negative way.

While it is often recommended, there is not sufficient research to draw any conclusions about the efficacy of family therapy for children or adolescents with depression. However, we would make the point that common sense argues that one family member's mood and behavior affects everyone in the family, and, at the very least, if everyone has an opportunity in a safe setting to express their emotions and gain some understanding about one another's feelings, that is a good thing. Also, having the entire family in therapy may help the child who is suffering from depression—if everyone is going to therapy, he may not feel so alone, so different.

Peer-to-peer group therapy is most often used in hospital settings or day programs where patients work together to solve common problems. It's a meeting-type format in which the therapist acts as a facilitator. It's usually used to address one particular issue, for example substance abuse, or to help children build and practice social skills. It's thought that these types of issues are more effectively addressed with one's peers than individually with one's therapist, though, again, there is not sufficient research to know whether it is an effective tool for either children or adolescents.

medications

The decision to use medication to treat your child's or adolescent's depression is a difficult one. The research is limited. The very subject matter is difficult to study—subjective symptoms like mood, thoughts and behavior don't easily lend themselves to objective measure.

Physicians prescribe a medication "off label" to a patient when they believe the medication will help alleviate symptoms, even though the medication hasn't been approved by the FDA for that particular illness or it hasn't been approved for use in the patient's age group. Ironically, "off label" prescribing occurs frequently for children and adolescents (for all medication, not just psychotropic medication) because of the ethical concerns about conducting studies on these age groups.

The studies don't tell us about either long term efficacy or safety of medication for children or teens. Although there are many medications to treat depression on the market, only one such medication, fluoxetine (brand name Prozac), has been approved by the FDA for use in children and adolescents, and most of the studies we have for children and adolescents focus solely on that medication. Physicians are often left with no option other than to prescribe medication "off-label."

All of this leaves physicians and parents with limited information (other than informed experience in the case of physicians) to help them make a decision about whether to treat a child's depression with medication and which medication to use. However, many mental health professionals and parents advocate for its use, particularly when talk therapy alone has been unsuccessful in treating depression or when a child is in imminent danger of hurting himself or someone else as a result of his depression.

FOUR
medications

CONSIDERING MEDICATION

Given all this, how do we, as parents, consider the options when thinking about giving our children medication to treat their depression? In the end, it boils down to trusting your child's psychiatrist, being as informed as you can, rigorously monitoring your child (both the taking of the medication and its effects and side effects) and keeping a bit of an open mind about both trying, adjusting or discontinuing the use of medication if benefits are not seen, or if the side effects are significant.

Most mental health professionals and The American Psychological Association, in its 2006 *Report of the Working Group on Psychotropic Medications for Children and Adolescents*, recommend a conservative approach when treating children and adolescents for depression—psychotherapy first, with regular monitoring, followed by carefully controlled medication (typically one of the SSRI antidepressants) together with the psychotherapy if the psychotherapy alone is not effective. If, however, your child is having significant difficulty with daily functioning, has particularly peculiar thinking, is focused on death, has attempted suicide or is engaging in other self-injurious behavior such as cutting, it may be best to begin with medication and psychotherapy as a combination treatment. If the situation is extremely dire—if your child is an immediate threat to himself or others or if he is hearing voices or seeing things that aren't there—you may need to consider hospitalization.

We now turn to the medication itself and some things you should know if you make the decision to begin medication.

BLACK BOX WARNING ON ANTIDEPRESSANTS.
One much-discussed side effect of antidepressant use is suicidal ideation (thinking about suicide). In 2004, the FDA issued a "black box warning" that the use of antidepressants in children, adolescents and young adults could lead to increased thoughts of suicide. It should be noted that while an increase in suicidal ideation did occur in the studies cited in the warning, in fact, no actual suicides occurred.

The warning reinforces the need for careful monitoring of antidepressant medication. If your child is prescribed an antidepressant, make sure that you and his psychiatrist are watching closely for signs of suicidal thinking or attempts.

TAKING MEDICATION

You should know that medication doesn't cure a mental disorder—it alleviates the symptoms, hopefully helping your child to function, participate in talk therapy, connect with other people, and ultimately recover from his episode.

Secondly, mood disorders like depression and bipolar disorder are complicated and our bodies are equally complicated. What works for one person doesn't work for another—it's the

rule rather than the exception that a lot of tweaking of psychotropic medication, both the type of medication and the dose, is required to find the one that works, in the dose that works. Several medications may be needed to fully address your child's disorder, or an additional medication may be needed to address the negative side effects of the first medication.

Children, adolescents and adults all metabolize medication differently. Younger people generally absorb medications into the blood stream more rapidly than older people do—this can cause higher peaking and more immediate side effects in children and adolescents than in adults. And younger people eliminate medications differently than adults do. A child's liver is proportionately larger than an adult's, so it eliminates medications more rapidly. Furthermore, many of these medications are absorbed into fat tissue before being released into the blood stream for use, which, especially for adolescent girls, can vary significantly over very short periods of time.

All of this means that the prescribing psychiatrist must consider a wide variety of factors when she chooses which medication and which dose best suits your child—and it means that there may be continuous need for adjustments before she finds the right medication and the right dose for your child. The general rule of thumb is to begin with the lowest dose possible, and then increase in small doses thereafter until the medication becomes effective.

Taking medication for mental disorders can be a pretty hard thing for your child—it can make him feel ashamed. It's important to establish an open attitude with your child about taking his medication. It may be helpful to compare taking psychotropic medication to taking medication for other kinds of medical problems, like an antibiotic for an ear infection, for example. You can tell your child that it's supposed to help him feel better (though it might take some time before it takes effect), and he deserves to do just that—feel better.

FOUR
medications

It's also pretty common for children and adolescents (and adults) to forget, unintentionally and sometimes intentionally, to take their medication, or to decide that they don't need it any more. This is particularly true once the medication begins to be effective. But withdrawal from these medications can be dangerous, so it's important that your child know how important it is to continue to take his medication on a daily basis, at the same time of day, and to continue his medication, even if he thinks he doesn't really need it. *A medication journal is very helpful in determining whether or not your child is taking his medication appropriately.*

Children should not be responsible for taking psychotropic medication and all children and adolescents should be monitored when they take psychotropic medication.

Withdrawal from psychotropic medication can be severe. You or your child should not make the unilateral decision to stop his medication. When it's time for your child to stop taking his medication, it is very important that your child taper down from using medication gradually, and under the supervision of his psychiatrist.

You can also check to make sure whether your child is taking his medication by keeping track of how many pills are in the bottle—if there are too many pills in it, then your child is not taking his medication. We should mention that it is not unheard of for children and adolescents to flush their medication down the toilet or otherwise dispose of it, or even sell or give it to others, so be careful about using the bottle check as your only evidence that your child is taking his medication. It's really best to have your child take his medication in your presence.

The problem of side effects can be an issue for your child. Many of the most common side effects—nausea, diarrhea, dry mouth, sleep disturbances, weight gain, the list can be long—occur shortly after beginning the medication and disappear within a few weeks. But some side effects are long term—often they can be managed by adjusting dosages or medications, but not always. The issue of side effects is further complicated by the age of your child—younger children may not be able to articulate what they are feeling.

Many psychotropic medications can be toxic and it's not always easy to tell what dose will be toxic for one person versus another. Some people inherently metabolize medications more slowly than others. In addition, several medications are sometimes required and the medications can interact with one another.

Some initial side effects, particularly suicidal ideation, can be dangerous. For that reason, it's important that your child see his psychiatrist frequently at the beginning of the process and whenever doses are adjusted or new medications are tried. **The FDA recommends that your child see his psychiatrist for regular monitoring once a week during the first month of treatment and every two weeks during the second month.** Regular monitoring, at least monthly, after that should occur.

The problem of long term side effects is a real issue. We don't know much about whether there are serious long-term side effects from even short-term use of psychotropic medication taken by children and adolescents. More research in this area is sorely needed.

Most psychotropic medications, antidepressant medications in particular, take time to work—up to four to six weeks—and even then relief from symptoms may be gradual. Furthermore, psychotropic medications tend to lose their effectiveness over time, so you may find that after a period of months, the medication that worked for your child no longer does and you have to go back to the drawing board. It can be frustrating for you and your child, but know that it is a normal part of using these medications.

Psychotropic medications can have a significant impact on other medications, even over-the-counter medications, being taken. Careful monitoring and complete disclosure to all of your child's physicians of medications (including over-the-counter medications, vitamins, herbal remedies and recreational drugs/alcohol) is a must. Most psychotropic medications should not be taken with alcohol or other recreational drugs; this issue should be thoroughly discussed with your child and his psychiatrist, **especially if your child has a history of alcohol or drug use.**

PSYCHOTROPIC MEDICATIONS

There are four classes of psychotropic medications used to treat mood disorders:
- antidepressants
- mood stabilizers
- antipsychotics
- antianxiety medications.

In general, antidepressants are by far the most used psychotropic medications and are used for the most common mood disorder—depression. Mood stabilizers are used for the treatment of bipolar disorder and sometimes as a secondary medication for depression. Antipsychotic medications are sometimes used to treat bipolar disorder or as short-term fast-acting medications for very severe episodes of depression. Antianxiety medications are used, as the name suggests, for the treatment of anxiety disorders—panic disorders, phobias, obsessive compulsive disorder (OCD), etc.—which often accompany depression.

FOUR
medications

Finally, though this is not a treatise on ADHD (attention deficit-hyperactivity disorder), we should mention the ADHD medications—particularly stimulants (Ritalin, Adderall, Concerta, etc.). Much is written, and debated, about the use of these medications. This handbook is not intended to address the complicated issue of ADHD, but we do recognize that many children with ADHD frequently also have other mental disorders, including depression. Given the complicated landscape of medications for both disorders, we can only advise you to make certain that any prescribing physician is aware of which medications your child is taking, and that she is qualified to understand the implications of simultaneously medicating your child for both disorders.

With this backdrop of information in mind, we will now discuss each of the classes of medications in more detail.

ANTIDEPRESSANTS

The most well known antidepressants are called re-uptake inhibitors. Re-uptake inhibitors have been around since the 1960s.

The first class of re-uptake inhibitors to be developed are called **tricyclic antidepressants**, TCAs (because of the three rings in their chemical structure). Tricyclics are not used much anymore because there are newer classes of re-uptake inhibitors with less severe side effects—overdoses of tricyclics can be very dangerous. However, they are still used occasionally, sometimes to treat ADHD, tic disorders, obsessive- compulsive disorder and bed-wetting in children and adolescents. In general, studies have shown that tricyclics are not effective for treating depression in children and adolescents.

A REMINDER: It's important that if your child is taking medication for his depression that he continue with his talk therapy. The two treatments complement one another. It's also important that the psychiatrist who prescribes the medication and the talk therapist communicate frequently so that appropriate adjustments can be made to your child's treatment plan. It is often up to the parent to make sure this happens—busy therapists often overlook this critical step in the process.

The newer, and most widely prescribed, class of antidepressants are generally known by their acronyms—**SSRI**s, **SARI**s, **SNRI**s, **NDRI**s. The most well known, and most used, are the SSRIs—selective serotonin re-uptake inhibitors. The other acronyms are usually referred to as second or third generation (or **atypical**) antidepressants. There are many of these medications on the market today and if your child needs medication to help him with his depression, he will probably begin with this class of antidepressants.

Only one antidepressant, the SSRI fluoxetine (Prozac) is approved by the FDA to treat depression in children and adolescents aged 8 and older. Many other antidepressants are used for children and teens, prescribed, as we mentioned before, "off-label."

Like most medications, antidepressants have side effects. Some are present during the first few weeks of taking the medication and then subside, and some are more persistent. The list is long and can include headache, nausea, gastrointestinal problems, diarrhea, constipation, vomiting, nervousness, agitation, skin rash, sleep problems, drowsiness, change in appetite, dizziness, irritability, blunting of emotions, weight gain, a feeling of being "wired" or over-stimulated and decreased sexual libido. Some side effects can be controlled through adjustment of the dosage, but some cannot.

On occasion, antidepressants, as with other psychotropic medications, can have the reverse effect—they exacerbate the depression that they are intended to alleviate. There are also reports that antidepressants may suppress growth, though this has not been confirmed.

Side effects vary significantly by individual and the only way to know which side effects your child may experience is informed trial and error, based on your child's psychiatrist's experience in general and with patients similar to your child.

Side effects and medical risks often increase when antidepressants are combined with other medications—in particular, negative interactions can occur when taking antidepressants with some antihistamines, antibiotics, blood pressure medications, stimulants, pain medications, sedatives and mood stabilizers.

Withdrawal from antidepressants can be difficult, including increased risk for manic episodes. Discontinuing their use requires tapering down the doses over a period of time and *must* be monitored by your child's psychiatrist.

FOUR
medications

Finally, we are again reminded that it's important to get a proper diagnosis when contemplating the use of an antidepressant for your child. Using antidepressants for people with bipolar disorder may provoke a manic episode or cause a spike in mood, leading to a bigger, potentially more dangerous drop afterward. It's very important to have an accurate diagnosis of your child's disorder and to be careful to note any unusual behaviors while taking antidepressants.

Another class of antidepressants works differently than those listed above. These antidepressants are called monoamine oxidase inhibitors (MAOIs). MAOIs have significant obstacles to use—many common foods interact dangerously with them—and so they are generally only used as a last line of defense for treating depression. MAOIs are not approved for use in children or adolescents.

MOOD STABILIZERS

Mood stabilizers, also called antimanic medications, are medications that even out, or stabilize, one's mood. They are used, often in conjunction with one another, to treat bipolar disorder and are sometimes used together with antidepressants to treat depression.

Be sure to ask your child's psychiatrist about the symptoms that signal toxic levels of lithium. The list is fairly long—you should be aware of them and call your child's psychiatrist immediately if any should develop.

One of the most commonly used mood stabilizers is lithium. It has been used for fifty years to treat bipolar disorder and a significant body of knowledge has grown up around it to help guide its administration and monitoring. Lithium is approved by the FDA for treating bipolar disorder in children aged 12 and older.

Lithium is extremely dose-sensitive, so it must be carefully administered and regularly monitored. It can adversely affect the thyroid and kidneys.

Lithium has a fairly wide range of side effects, particularly when first taking it, including restlessness, mental slowing, drowsiness, weakness, fatigue, nausea, diarrhea, gastrointestinal problems, hair loss or thinning, weight gain, tremors, acne flare-ups, hypothyroidism, dry mouth, excessive thirst, water retention and increased urination (including bed-wetting in children). Many of these side effects can be managed by adjusting the dosage. Longer term side effects can include weakened bones, weight gain, hypothyroidism and kidney damage. In addition, birth defects are associated with the use of lithium if used during pregnancy and caution should be taken when using lithium during breast-feeding.

Because of the way lithium works in the body, sodium levels are important—both significant increases and decreases can be dangerous. If your child is taking lithium, he should be careful not to increase or reduce his sodium intake excessively—even drinking too much or too little water, sweating, vomiting or diarrhea, the use of diuretics, or crash dieting can be dangerous. Also, you should be careful about the regular use of some anti-inflammatory agents (such as ibuprofen) and excessive intake of caffeine when taking lithium.

The other mood stabilizers that are used to treat mood disorders are the group of medications known as anticonvulsants. Because of the dose-sensitivity of lithium, and because lithium does not work for everyone, this class of medications, originally designed to prevent seizures, is being used more and more as an alternative to lithium.

The anticonvulsant valproate, divalproex or valproic acid is the most commonly used anticonvulsant medication to treat bipolar disorder—used probably as much as lithium, especially to treat rapid-cycling bipolar disorder.

As with other psychotropic medications, valproate has a long list of potential side effects. Initial side effects can include gastrointestinal upset, headache, dizziness, double vision, anxiety, confusion and sleepiness. More long-lasting side effects are increased appetite, weight gain, tremors and hair loss. In addition, there is a chance of birth defects associated with the use of valproate during pregnancy and caution should be taken when using it during breast-feeding. Valproate can also cause cessation of menstruation, excess facial and body hair and ovarian cysts in teenage girls and women.

The dosage of this medication varies greatly from person to person depending on metabolism rates—regular monitoring is required to check for liver and pancreatic toxicity. Talk to your child's psychiatrist about the symptoms that signal toxicity.

Valproate has not been approved by the FDA for use in children or adolescents for bipolar disorder, though it has been approved to treat bipolar disorder in adults.

There are other anticonvulsants though they are used less frequently than lithium and valproate. As with other psychotropic medication, the side effects of these medications can be significant. None have been approved for use in children and adolescents. Regular monitoring should be done to check for toxicity.

ANTIPSYCHOTICS

If your child is having a particularly severe episode of depression, has delusions or hallucinations, or is in need of hospitalization, you may find yourself being asked to consider an antipsychotic medication. Because antipsychotic drugs act rapidly to relieve symptoms, they are used to bridge the gap between the onset of taking an antidepressant and when it begins to take effect.

Antipsychotics are also used as a stand-alone medication to treat bipolar disorder in children and adolescents if other medications have failed to be effective and are also sometimes used early on to level out a manic episode until a mood stabilizer takes effect.

Like re-uptake inhibitors, antipsychotic drugs have gone through a generation since their discovery in the 1950s. The class of antipsychotic drugs used today is called "atypical antipsychotics." These medications have not been approved by the FDA for children younger than 18.

If your child is asked to take an antipsychotic medication, it's a good idea to do some research on the specific type of medication he is being asked to take. The side effects, especially the long-term ones, of these medications can be serious, and include increased risk of diabetes and cardiovascular disease (both of which should be monitored for regularly). Your child's psychiatrist and research on the Internet can give you specific information about the risks and benefits of these medications. We have a listing of several on-line resources at the end of this chapter.

ANTIANXIETY MEDICATIONS

If your child suffers from an anxiety disorder, he may be asked to take an antianxiety medication. While antidepressants can be effective to treat anxiety disorders and are often used to do so, antianxiety medications are specifically designed to treat anxiety, and they relieve symptoms quickly.

Antianxiety medications include benzodiazepines. Their side effects include sleepiness, loss of coordination, fatigue and mental slowing. For some people, these medications can have the opposite effect—they can increase anxiety rather than relieve it.

These drugs can be habit-forming—abuse of them can easily occur and sudden withdrawal can be dangerous. Because of this, they are most often used on a temporary or an as-needed basis. These medications have not been approved for use in children younger than 18 years old.

The other drug used to treat anxiety and sometimes as a secondary medication for depression is buspirone. It is not a fast-acting medication, cannot be taken on an as-needed basis as can benzodiazepines, and is not generally as effective as benzodiazepines—but it does not have the same risk of addiction or dependence. Side effects include dizziness, drowsiness, nausea, headache and nervousness. Buspirone has not been approved for use in children and adolescents under the age of 18.

MORE INFORMATION ON MEDICATION

This section on medication has been only a starter for you. There is much more information you will want to ask your child's psychiatrist about—she should be able to answer many, if not all, of your questions.

Information about psychotropic medications changes relatively frequently. It's a good idea to check with your child's psychiatrist from time to time to see whether there is any new information that would suggest discontinuance of your child's medication or whether there is any reason to believe that a different medication might be more effective for your child. You may also want to ask to see the research or to read about it online.

In addition, there is a plethora of information on the Internet—of course the usual precautions should be taken when relying on information you get from the Internet, but here are some websites you may want to refer to:

- *Drugs.com*
- The Food and Drug Administration (*www.fda.gov*)
- *Mayoclinic.org*
- *Medlineplus.gov*
- *Pdrhealth.com*

FOUR
medications

brain stimulation therapies

Brain simulation therapies are exactly what they sound like—therapies that stimulate specific parts of the brain. Some, like ECT, have been around a long time and some are new. If you are considering one of these therapies, you may wish to consult with your child's therapist and physician before researching the options available. Following is a summary of some of the brain stimulation therapies currently being used, although this field is an ever changing one.

Neurofeedback is a form of biofeedback in which the patient retrains his brain waves. Electrodes are attached to the patient's scalp. A therapist "reads" the patient's brain waves via the electrodes and gives feedback to the patient. The patient then can use this feedback to re-wire the brain. There are mixed views on whether or not neurofeedback is effective in treating depression.

ECT therapy (electroconvulsive therapy) is the most researched and longest used of the brain stimulation therapies. It has been shown to be an effective treatment for severe depression or bipolar disorder when talk therapy and medication have not been effective, or when a patient is not responding to the outside world (catatonia), is suicidal, or is malnourished as a result of his disorder.

The patient is put under anesthesia, electrodes are applied to the patient's scalp and electrical currents are passed through the patient's brain, causing a seizure that lasts for less than a minute. Because the patient is under anesthesia, no pain or discomfort is experienced by the patient. Treatment consists of sessions a few times a week for somewhere between two and four weeks, with possible maintenance sessions thereafter. A patient undergoing ECT will often continue taking medication in addition to the ECT.

Vagus (or vagal) nerve stimulation (VNS) involves implanting a pacemaker-like device in the patient's chest and connecting the device via wiring to the left vagus nerve located at the base of the brain. The pulse generator sends electrical pulses to the vagus nerve, which sends these signals to the brain. VNS has been approved by the FDA for treatment of depression in patients who have long-term, severe or recurrent depression that has not responded to at least four other treatments. Though approved by the FDA, research about its effectiveness is mixed.

Repetitive transcranial magnetic stimulation (rTMS or TMS) is a treatment in which magnets are placed near the area of the patient's brain that is involved in mood regulation. Short electromagnetic pulses are then administered, causing small electrical currents that stimulate

the nerve cells in the targeted area. rTMS/TMS is used in patients who have not responded to at least one antidepressant medication and is sometimes used instead of ECT. rTMS is approved by the FDA but research about its effectiveness is mixed.

Magnetic seizure therapy (MST) borrows from both ECT and rTMS. It uses a magnet, like rTMS, to stimulate the brain, but at a higher frequency in order to induce a seizure, like ECT. Like ECT, the patient is anesthetized during the procedure. MST is in the early stages of testing.

Deep brain stimulation (DBS) is an experimental treatment requiring surgery in which a pair of electrodes is implanted in the brain, and, like rTMS, contolled by a pulse generator implanted in the chest. DBS is only available on an experimental basis at this time.

FIVE
brain
stimulation
therapies

FOR MORE INFORMATION about brain stimulation therapies, go to
http://www.nimh.nih.gov/health/topics/brain-stimulation-therapies/brain-stimulation-therapies.shtml

supplements, mind-body therapies and other therapies

When it comes to mental disorders like depression, there is a plethora of alternative treatments available, almost jumping out at you, to consider. Some of them are silly, and some are commonsensical. Some will seem too good to be true—and probably are. This chapter is written to give you a very general sense of some of the alternatives being discussed today.

SUPPLEMENTS

St. John's wort and Sam-e may help relieve the symptoms of depression. There is some evidence that omega-3 fatty acids (found in fish oil, flax, walnuts) may help with milder forms of depression. There is also some suggestion that B vitamins and Vitamin D may be helpful.

Make sure your child is using any of these supplements under the care of a physician, and that, if your child is taking psychotropic medication, your child's prescribing physician or psychiatrist know of, and approves, your child's taking of any of these supplements. St. John's wort can interact negatively with antidepressants and can decrease the effectiveness of oral contraceptives and Sam-e can trigger mania in people with bipolar disorder.

MIND-BODY THERAPIES

Many people experiment successfully with yoga, tai chi, meditation, breathing exercises, guided imagery, acupuncture, massage, relaxation techniques and full-spectrum light therapy to relieve or manage their symptoms of depression. Some therapists recommend these therapies as adjunct therapies to talk therapy and medication. And there is some compelling evidence that meditation may be particularly helpful—studies show that meditation literally changes the brain. People who meditate show physical increases in the size of and activity in the part of the cortex associated with emotions.

The Center for Investigating Healthy Minds (*www.investigatinghealthyminds.org*) at the University of Wisconsin has more information about the research being done on the benefits of mind/body therapies as well as a list of other resources.

SmilingMind (*www.smilingmind.com.au*) is a website and app that has meditation practices for all age groups, including children, pre-teens and teenagers. There are many other websites and apps available to help you begin a meditation practice as well.

OTHER THERAPIES

And, as we all know, you will find many other treatments by even a quick search of the Internet. As we said before, some of these treatments may be tempting. We can only say that it's important to talk to your child's physician and therapist before trying alternative treatments to make sure they are not harmful, especially if your child is taking psychotropic medication.

In addition, be wary of quick fixes—they are likely not supported by research, and may even be scams. It's wise to thoroughly research any alternative you want to try.

SIX
supplements,
mind-body
therapies
and other
therapies

strategies for good mental health

We all want good mental—and physical—health, but how do we attain, and then keep, it? We live in a world that constantly places stresses on us, stresses that can have an impact on our bodies and our minds. So, what can we do to lessen the impact of stress and increase our capacity for good mental health? Here are a few ideas.

Exercise. Lots of research supports the benefits of exercise, both for our physical but also for our mental health. Try to aim for 30 minutes daily or 2.5 hours weekly of moderate exercise.

Nutrition. The brain needs the same vitamins and minerals, proteins, healthy carbohydrates and good fats that the body does in order to support its healthy functioning, and just like the body, the brain reacts poorly to excess amounts of things like sugar, alcohol and drugs. Try to maintain a healthy diet. If you are having trouble managing your diet, keep a food journal. It may help you better monitor your diet and adjust it to be a healthier one. Of course, like everything, don't beat yourself up if it isn't always perfect. No one's is. Good enough is good enough.

Sleep. We live in a sleep deprived society. Research says that we need at least 8 hours of sleep a night, and children and teens need more than that. Good sleep habits are important to a good night's sleep. Try to observe regular sleep hours in a cool, dark, quiet environment. Adopting a bedtime ritual like a warm shower or bath, reading a book or listening to quiet music can be helpful. It's important to limit activities that stimulate the brain—talking to friends on the phone and using screens that are backlit are impediments to getting a good night's sleep.

Sun. Admit it, you feel better when the sun is shining, don't you? There is a reason for that—we need sun. Getting plenty of sunshine has been correlated with improved mental health. Get it when you can!

ONE
strategies
for good
mental health

Avoid substances that are harmful. Drugs, alcohol, excessive amount of sugar—these things are not good for the body, and definitely not good for the mind. Children and teens in particular should not use drugs or alcohol—their brains are still developing and both drugs and alcohol can make long term changes in the brains.

Manage activities that are stressful. Of course, we can't avoid all things that are stressful in life, but we can manage at least some activities that are stressful. The first thing to do is to identify those things that make you feel stressed. You can then work to manage those situations—eliminate them altogether if you can, spend as little time doing them as possible, prepare and recover from them by doing something that relaxes you before and after, or talk to a trusted friend or advisor about the situations and brainstorm ways of dealing with them. These seemingly simple ideas can help you reduce the overall stress in your daily life.

Do more activities that are not stressful. What do you like to do? Paint? Read? Spend more time with friends? Listen to music? Do more of it!

Practice gratitude. Gratitude is a thankful appreciation of what you have in life and an acknowledgement of the good in life, including the good qualities of others. In research, gratitude is strongly and consistently associated with greater optimism, happiness and a greater sense of belonging. It helps you focus on what you have, instead of what you lack. Research also shows that you can foster gratitude by practicing it—people who kept a gratitude journal, writing a few sentences a week, were more optimistic and felt better about their lives.

Gratitude turns what we have into enough.

Take a personal inventory. Ask yourself the following questions:
- What are three strengths of mine?
- What are three things I'd like to work on?
- When I get stressed, how do I cope?
- What are some positive coping strategies I could do that I don't currently do?

Be mindful. Mindfulness is being present in the moment, paying attention to what is going on around you, without multi-tasking and without thinking about the past or what you have to do later today, tomorrow or next week. It seems evident that when are more mindful, we are less stressed—we spend less time trying to do two things at once, or thinking about all of the things that we are not getting done—we are happier in the moment. Although it's probably not possible to be always 100% mindful, trying to approach life from a more mindful perspective can help reduce the effects of stress on our minds and bodies.

Meditate. There is now quite a bit of research that tells us that meditation is good for our minds and bodies. People who meditate have observable changes in their brains, and consistently report being happier than those who do not meditate. It only take a few minutes a day to incorporate a meditation practice into your life.

Care for others. Current research on happiness tells us that caring for others is a necessary component to happiness and good mental health. Both close personal relationships and altruistic acts have been shown to give meaning to our lives and increase our sense of happiness and well-being.

There are many more ways of fostering and maintaining good mental health. You can check out the many websites dedicated to happiness and mindfulness for more ideas. In the meantime, try practicing even some of the ideas above, and we wish you all the best in your pursuit of good mental health.

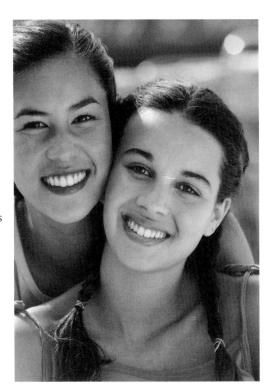

happiness

There is now a group of psychologists who are studying, not mental disorders, but mental health—their research asks the question: **what does it take to make one happy?** Their answer? Three things:

- Strong, meaningful relationships
- A purpose to one's life
- Setting and achieving goals towards that purpose.

In their very simplicity, there is much to contemplate.

Though our handbook has been about depression and how to deal with it if your child is suffering from it, in some ways this handbook relates to the question of happiness. The underlying intention of the book is the same intention we give every day to raising our children—not just providing them with food, clothing and shelter, but providing them with a firm basis on which to stand as adults and achieve their own happiness.

As you travel the road that many of us have been down before, keep in mind that your ultimate goal is this goal too—the happiness of your child—and that it's the goal of every single parent, from time immemorial to the present second and beyond. We are all connected to one another in this very meaningful endeavor.

The Positive Psychology Center at the University of Pennsylvania (www.ppc.sas.upenn.edu) is a great resource if you want to know more about the field of Positive Psychology.

A CONCLUDING LETTER

It has been said that it takes a village to raise a child, and this handbook is our attempt to be a virtual village for you, to help at a particularly difficult time in your lives—a time when you might feel like there is no village out there for you.

If you need more information, there are many websites available on the Internet, and some good reference books available for purchase or at your local library.

And while we've tried to be as accurate, complete and objective as we could in our handbook, please remember that we are parents—not professionals dispensing either medical or psychological advice. You should rely on your child's professionals for that.

We wish you and your family all the best. We welcome your comments and suggestions. Please write to us at Post Office Box 616, Winnetka, Illinois 60093 or email us at *info@erikaslighthouse.org*.

Sincerely,
The Board of Directors
Erika's Lighthouse
April 2016

Pay it forward, pass it on … Just as we are passing this information along to you, we hope you will do the same. If you have a friend or neighbor in need of this handbook, please tell her that she can download or purchase a copy by visiting our website. And … thank you.

about Erika's Lighthouse

Erika's Lighthouse: A Beacon of Hope for Adolescent Depression was founded in 2004 by Virginia and Thomas Neuckranz after their daughter Erika lost her life to depression. Tom and Ginny founded Erika's Lighthouse to be a beacon of hope for the many other young people who struggle with depression, empowering them with the knowledge and skills to understand and cope with this and other mental disorders.

Erika's Lighthouse educates communities about childhood and teen depression, helps eliminate the stigma associated with mental disorders like depression and empowers our youth to maintain good mental health.

TO DOWLOAD FOR FREE OR TO PURCHASE AN E-BOOK OR A PRINTED COPY of the *Parent Handbook on Childhood and Teen Depression*, please go to *www.erikaslighthouse.org*.

TO JOIN OUR MAILING LIST for news and information about Erika's Lighthouse, please go to *www.erikaslighthouse.org* or email us at *info@erikaslighthouse.org*.

TO MAKE A TAX-DEDUCTIBLE DONATION to Erika's Lighthouse, please go to *www.erikaslighthouse.org* or make your check payable to Erika's Lighthouse and mail it to us at Erika's Lighthouse, Post Office Box 616, Winnetka, Illinois 60093. Thank you!